Pers

The *Essential Clinical Skills for Nurses* series focuses on key clinical skills for nurses and other health professionals. These concise, accessible books assume no prior knowledge and focus on core clinical skills, clearly presenting common clinical procedures and their rationale, together with the essential background theory. Their user-friendly format makes them an indispensable guide to clinical practice for all nurses, especially to student nurses and newly qualified staff.

Other titles in the *Essential Clinical Skills for Nurses* series:

Personal Hygiene Care

Lindsay Dingwall
School of Nursing and Midwifery
University of Dundee
Ninewells Hospital
Dundee
UK

⊛WILEY-BLACKWELL

A John Wiley & Sons, Ltd., Publication

This edition first published 2010
© 2010 Lindsay Dingwall

Blackwell Publishing was acquired by John Wiley & Sons in February 2007.
Blackwell's publishing programme has been merged with Wiley's global
Scientific, Technical, and Medical business to form Wiley-Blackwell.

Registered office
John Wiley & Sons Ltd, The Atrium, Southern Gate, Chichester,
West Sussex, PO19 8SQ, United Kingdom

Editorial offices
9600 Garsington Road, Oxford, OX4 2DQ, United Kingdom
2121 State Avenue, Ames, Iowa 50014-8300, USA

For details of our global editorial offices, for customer services and for information about how to apply for permission to reuse the copyright material in
this book please see our website at www.wiley.com/wiley-blackwell.

The right of the author to be identified as the author of this work has been
asserted in accordance with the Copyright, Designs and Patents Act 1988.

Wiley also publishes its books in a variety of electronic formats. Some
content that appears in print may not be available in electronic books.

Designations used by companies to distinguish their products are often
claimed as trademarks. All brand names and product names used in this
book are trade names, service marks, trademarks or registered trademarks of
their respective owners. The publisher is not associated with any product or
vendor mentioned in this book. This publication is designed to provide
accurate and authoritative information in regard to the subject matter
covered. It is sold on the understanding that the publisher is not engaged in
rendering professional services. If professional advice or other expert assistance is required, the services of a competent professional should be sought.

Library of Congress Cataloging-in-Publication Data

Dingwall, Lindsay.
Personal hygiene care / Lindsay Dingwall.
p. ; cm. – (Essential clinical skills for nurses series)
Includes bibliographical references and index.
ISBN 978-1-4051-6307-1 (pbk. : alk. paper) 1. Nursing. 2. Patients–
Care. 3. Patients–Health and hygiene. I. Title. II. Series: Essential
clinical skills for nurses.
[DNLM: 1. Hygiene. 2. Nursing Care–methods. WY 100 D584p
2010]

RT42.D56 2010
610.73–dc22
2009040322

A catalogue record for this book is available from the British Library.

Set in 9/11.5 pt Palatino by Toppan Best-set Premedia Limited
Printed and bound in Malaysia by KHL Printing Co Sdn Bhd

1   2010

Contents

Preface

Feeling fresh and clean is something most of us take for granted. We can usually choose the products we prefer and follow our own routines for showering or bathing and general grooming. Often if we cannot manage to wash, clean our teeth or wash our hair, we can become very aware that we perhaps don't look our best and this can lead us to not feel our best. People who are ill or unable to wash and groom themselves are no different – looking and feeling clean and cared for is important for them to feel their best too.

Fundamental patient care – meeting the personal care needs of the patients – is the aspect of nursing which patients need for comfort and confidence. Like us, no patient has exactly the same washing routines and preferences; unlike many of us, patients may depend on others to carry out these essential needs.

This book aims to help you to understand some of these needs and to be able to carry out nursing procedures covering all aspects of personal hygiene. Chapter 1 outlines some of the issues which should be thought about before, during and after the procedures. The emphasis is on assessing the patient. Assessment merely means gathering all the information needed to carry out care safely to meet an individual's preferences and requirements. This may be assessing risk, for example allergies; it may be about assessing what help they may require; or it may be about assessing what influence aspects of their life have on personal cleansing, for example religion, age or ability to understand and contribute to the skill.

Personal cleansing is one of the activities of living (i.e. the activities we undertake every day that are often taking them for granted, e.g. walking, eating and breathing). Chapter 1 asks you to think about how not being able to carry out one activity can impact on the other activities. For example, if a patient finds it difficult to breathe easily, this may make it difficult to walk or take a bath. Planning care with the patient should take into account their activities of living. You will see that core elements of each skill include explaining to the patient what the procedure will entail, gaining their informed consent (meaning that the patient understands and agrees to the procedure) and planning with the patient how they can contribute. The importance of evaluating whether the nursing care has been successful is also discussed in Chapter 1. If care has been successful, the patients will have had their needs met in a manner with which they are happy and that will contribute to their general health and well-being.

How to carry out the care is identified in the different skills outlined throughout the chapters. Each chapter looks at a different aspect of personal hygiene and provides a brief overview of the anatomy of the part of the body being focused on. Some influences on the patient's health are discussed, for example what may cause patients to have poor oral health and how to recognise some of the common conditions.

Some of the skills described will help to identify risks to the patients' health; others describe how to meet the everyday needs of patients safely.

Overall, this book is intended to help you to meet patients' personal hygiene needs and preferences and to help you to think about how to meet each patient's individual needs.

The skills associated with personal hygiene may not be the highly technical skills that might have become valued in nursing, but they are essential to the patient.

Lindsay Dingwall

Acknowledgements

Chapter 4's figures of hearing aids were used with the kind permission of Oticon Ltd (registered office: Victoria House, Brighton Road, Redhill, Surrey RH1 6QZ).

Many thanks to Wiley-Blackwell for their kind permission to allow use of anatomical images throughout the book.

Thanks to Jessica Ballantine for her tact and diplomacy and help with finishing the book.

Thank you especially to Nick, Ewan and Callum for their patience at home and to kind colleagues (Kate, Robert, Michelle and Fiona) for their encouragement at work.

In memory of my husband
Andy Dingwall (1956–2009)
Loved always

Assessing Your Patient

1

INTRODUCTION

This chapter is intended to illustrate why maintaining the personal hygiene needs of patients is so important. General principles of assessment will be identified relating to the patient's normal living routines, safety of the patient and the care environment. More specific assessment and nursing interventions to meet specific hygiene needs, such as ear care or oral hygiene, will be introduced throughout each chapter.

The aim of this chapter is to help the reader understand the role of general comprehensive nursing assessment in meeting personal hygiene needs.

LEARNING OUTCOMES

After reading this chapter, the reader will be able to:

❏ Discuss the principles of assessment for individualising patient care, including the use of assessment tools.
❏ Identify infection control measures which require to be assessed.
❏ Outline the health and safety issues which require assessment before agreeing nursing interventions.
❏ Discuss the importance of assessing the environment before meeting hygiene needs.
❏ Describe assessment measures while carrying out prescribed care.
❏ Discuss the role of evaluating nursing interventions and the role of documentation.

THE IMPORTANCE OF PERSONAL HYGIENE IN GENERAL PATIENT CARE

Any person who is unable to meet their own hygiene needs risks not only feeling psychologically worse but also deteriorating physically.

Historically, good patient hygiene has been seen as important for preventing the spread of disease. The skin is the first defence against disease and there is evidence that keeping the skin clean reduces the number of microorganisms, for example bacteria that can cause the spread of infection (Horton & Parker, 2002).

However, other benefits to the patient should be considered: looking and feeling clean is important for a patient's feeling of well-being and confidence to interact socially.

When we are no longer able to initiate our own personal hygiene at a time of our choosing and in the manner we prefer, our feeling of social and psychological well-being is reduced (Switzer, 2001). For some people even the motivation to meet their hygiene needs can reduce as the process becomes more difficult. This may be for many reasons: the impact of illness, mobility difficulties, pain, psychological distress or embarrassment at requiring intimate care from a stranger.

The practice of assisting a person to meet their hygiene needs as well as helping the patient can develop the nurse–patient relationship and allows a skilled practitioner to assess how the patient is progressing physically and mentally. Any changes to the patient's physical condition and ability or their mood can be noted and acted upon. Of equal importance is the role that meeting a person's hygiene needs in terms of skin, hair and nail care has in promoting individualised care and dignity.

Nursing staff have a duty to meet the fundamental needs of patients under their care; however, according to the Healthcare Commission (2007), around 30% of the complaints received about hospital care relate to nurses not meeting the patients' basic needs, such as personal hygiene or nutrition. Indeed, the Department of Health (DH; 2000) reached consensus in its document *No Secrets* that 'acts of neglect or omission' constitute abuse of vulnerable adults. These include ignoring physical or medical needs, failing to provide access to appropriate healthcare services and withholding necessities. Personal hygiene, including washing and oral health, is included among these necessities. The *Essence of Care* (Department of Health, 2001) outlines the need for healthcare staff – and nurses in particular – to meet the fundamental needs of patients in care. Personal and oral hygiene are among the areas of care particularly focused on in this document.

Nursing staff, however, are not the sole healthcare professionals involved in assisting patients to maintain their hygiene needs. Box 1.1 illustrates an example of some other healthcare professionals and allied health professionals who may also be involved, as well as the patient's family should the patient wish.

A SYSTEMATIC APPROACH TO MEETING PATIENT NEEDS

At any time the patients in care will be diverse in terms of age, ability, culture and physical and mental abilities; certain patient

---

Box 1.1 Other health professionals who may be involved in meeting patients' hygiene needs

- Specialist nurses, e.g. tissue viability nurses/continence nurses/diabetes specialists.
- Liaison nurses, e.g. mental health/child nurses/learning disability nurses.
- General medical staff/general practitioners.
- Specialist medical staff, e.g. dermatologists; orthotics and prosthetics; ear, nose and throat.
- Primary healthcare staff.
- Hospital/community pharmacists.
- Opticians.
- Audiologists.
- Podiatrists.
- Occupational therapists.
- Physiotherapists.
- Dentists.
- Dental hygienists.
- Speech and language therapists.
- Dieticians.

> **Box 1.2 Patient populations likely to require assistance in meeting hygiene needs**
>
> The very old and very young.
> People with learning disabilities.
> People with cognitive difficulties, i.e. difficulty understanding.
> People with physical difficulties.
> People with mental health problems.
> People undergoing chemotherapy and radiotherapy.
> People prescribed medication affecting oral or skin health.
> People with fluctuating consciousness levels.
> People who require 'end of life' care (terminally ill).

populations are more likely to have particular difficulty in meeting their own hygiene needs (Box 1.2).

However, an individual patient's ability to self-care may also vary on a daily basis or even more frequently within a period of admission. For example, a patient may be independent before an operation but may take several days post-surgery to reach this level again; a patient may react badly to medication and become too confused to manage independently for some time and a patient who is undergoing a period of rehabilitation after a stroke may take several weeks to reach the level where they can self-care. Therefore, hygiene needs must be evaluated and reassessed whenever a patient's condition improves or deteriorates (Ashurst, 2003) and the nurse must be responsive to the continual changes in the needs and concerns of each patient.

In order to treat each patient as an individual, the nursing process or systematic approach to nursing is used in the majority of healthcare situations in Britain.

Identified as the core and essence of nursing (Pope *et al.*, 1995), the nursing process ensures that nurses employ a logical, systematic and rational approach towards care delivery. Where possible, the patient should have an active and equal role in the nursing process unless physical or emotional limitations reduce their ability to participate. Therefore, the patient is placed at the centre of the care process and, in conjunction with the patient's continu-

Table 1.1 Components of the nursing process and associated nursing activities

Nursing process components	Nursing process activities
Assessment stage	• Collect and organise data (information) from and about the patient • Validate (check) data • Document data (in care records)
Nursing diagnosis stage	• Analyse data • Identify problems • Identify patient's strengths and weaknesses • Devise statements which reflect the problem • Document problem statements
Planning stage	• Prioritise patient's problems • Decide goals and expected care outcomes with the patient • Identify the interventions required to meet goals • Formulate the patient care plan
Implementation/ intervention stage	• Implement the interventions • Assist the patient towards self-care if possible • Document nursing/patient activity
Evaluation/ reassessment stage	• Review the patient's progress in relation to meeting goals • Collect and review data • Reassess the patient and modify care plan if needs are not met

ous input regarding their condition, the nurse will use a problem-solving approach in order to meet the needs of the patient.

The nursing process comprises five components, or stages, which are followed in order. The process is also cyclical, that is using the process requires the nurse to assess, follow the stages and reassess throughout the patient's care episode. Table 1.1 illustrates the components and the activities carried out under these headings (Holland, 2008; Kozier *et al.*, 2008).

Using the nursing process ensures patient-centred care of a high quality and that clinically effective care is carried out. The cornerstone of the nursing process is nursing assessment where the patient's own particular care needs are identified (Hamilton & Price, 2007).

Nursing assessment

The purpose of nursing assessment is to collect and process data (information) about the patient in order to develop a clear picture about the patient and his/her needs. Assessment therefore has to be 'holistic' in that all aspects of the patient's life are assessed and not only the physical aspects of their condition (Table 1.2). The components of holistic assessment are discussed in more detail later in this chapter.

Table 1.2 Components and examples of holistic assessment

Components of holistic assessment	Examples of assessment questions relating to personal hygiene
Physical: the patient's ability to self-care; the effect of the disease process on the body/organs	Is the patient physically able to manage their own hygiene needs?
	What interventions will be required by the nurse?
	Does the patient have any allergies, e.g. to soap?
	Does the patient require any prescribed preparations, e.g. bath additives, medicated shampoo, skin preparations?
Psychological: the patient's mental state; the effects of any disease process; the effect of illness/admission on the patient's mental health.	Does the patient have any mental health condition which will interfere with their understanding of carrying out hygiene needs safely?
	Does the patient have any anxieties or fears about aspects of personal hygiene?
	Does the patient recognise the need to maintain personal hygiene?
Sociological	Are there any factors which may hinder a patient's ability to meet their hygiene needs?
	Do the patient's home circumstances affect their ability to self-care?
Spiritual	Does the patient have any religious beliefs that must be taken into account when meeting hygiene needs?
	Are there any factors relating to hygiene which may affect the patient's well-being and/or relationships?
Cultural	Does the patient hold specific beliefs about meeting hygiene needs that must be taken account of?
	Does the patient express a preference for same-sex nursing care?

Data can be objective, that is measured (e.g. temperature or urine output) or seen/felt/smelled (e.g. the nurse may smell that a patient has been unable to meet their own hygiene needs) or subjective, that is what the patient feels (e.g. pain or fear of falling while having a shower).

Assessment on admission or at the beginning of a care episode helps the nurse to establish a baseline of the patient's condition. Having a clear baseline allows the nurse to measure any subsequent improvement or deterioration in the patient's condition. For example, assessing a patient's ability to wash at the first opportunity allows the nurse to decide at a later date whether the patient's ability is improving.

Assessment at the initial stage of admission to care is also vital to identify any risk to the patient, other patients in the clinical area or healthcare staff. For example, patient allergies can be determined and the level of mobility and mobility aids used can be assessed, as can the risks of infection and pressure sores.

Data can be sourced from many people. The patient is the most direct source of data; however, not all patients will be able to supply the information required to safely proceed with nursing care. The patient may be too young to understand/answer questions or may be too ill to respond. In these types of circumstances, secondary sources of information should be explored. These may be the relatives or carers of the patient, other healthcare professionals known to the patient (e.g. the general practitioner or community nurse) or staff from other hospital departments (e.g. the admissions department). Documentation can be useful in relaying information about a patient (e.g. nursing care plan, doctor's referral letter or transfer letter from a different care setting). Interaction with the patient also provides a clear opportunity for nursing assessment using a range of nursing skills (Box 1.3).

The data gathered about the patient should be documented in the patient's care plan as evidence of the decision-making process and to inform other members of the healthcare team.

Box 1.3 Nursing skills required for nursing assessment

- Utilising the five senses: sight, touch, hearing, smell and (to a lesser extent) taste.
- Communication skills: to establish a relationship with the patient and to access as much information as possible and to assist the patient through the nursing process as an active partner.
- Observation skills: to determine aspects of what the patient may not feel able/ be able to tell you.
- Measurement skills: to enable the nurse to use screening and risk assessment tools effectively; to evaluate the effects of care.
- Clinical skills: to enable the nurse to be able to carry out the assessment process safely and accurately.
- Critical thinking skills: to enable the nurse to make sense of the data and to be able to prioritise care requirements.
- The skills to apply theory to clinical care. This enables the nurse to use their knowledge in establishing reasons for care needs and to educate the patient.

Scenario 1.1

Mrs Jones, an 82-year-old female patient, has been admitted as an emergency to your clinical area after being found by a neighbour after a fall at home. She has no relatives or other carers accompanying her and there is little written information available. She has told you during the initial assessment interview that she has no problems with mobility, washing and eating. You are unsure as to whether she has been able to provide you with a full picture of how she has been coping. You are walking with her to the area in your ward where the weighing scales are kept.

Think about how you can use the nursing skills required for assessment to establish more information for her baseline assessment during the walk to the weighing scales.

Suggestions for Scenario 1.1

While walking with the patient you can use:

- Observation skills: assess Mrs Jones' mobility
  - Is she steady on her feet?
  - How quickly can she manage to walk?
  - Does she appear to be in pain?
  - Can she use her mobility aid correctly (if used)?
  - Would she benefit from a physiotherapy referral?

- Observation skills: assess Mrs Jones' teeth and speech
  - Can she speak clearly?
  - Do her teeth appear to be clean?
  - Does she have dentures?
  - Do they appear to be a good fit?
- Observation/sight/touch/smell: assess Mrs Jones' skin
  - Does her skin appear thin and/or dry?
  - Could she be dehydrated?
  - Does her skin feel dry or papery to the touch?
  - Does her skin look clean?
  - Are there any signs of injury or skin conditions?
- Communication skills
  - Can she maintain a conversation?
  - Does her sight appear to be normal?
  - Is her hearing normal?
  - Does the patient appear to understand your conversation?
- Observations skills: assessing Mrs Jones' nutrition
  - Do her clothes appear loose?
  - Does she appear to be lighter/smaller than her weight?
- Observation skills/sight/smell: assessing Mrs Jones' hygiene
  - Are her clothes clean?
  - Does her hair look washed and care for?
  - Are her nails clean?
  - Does she smell fresh?
  - Is there any evidence of elimination problems?

These observations allow the nurse to use critical thinking skills and theoretical knowledge to pursue any discrepancies with the patient. Gentle questioning and good communication skills can allow the nurse to explore these with the patient and to find out why the patient may be reluctant to disclose problems to the nurse.

Screening as part of assessment

The terms 'screening' and 'assessment' have become so confused as to be used interchangeably, but in fact they are two discrete nursing approaches (Mousley, 2006). Screening could be defined as a 'public health service in which members of a defined population, who do not necessarily perceive they are at risk of, or are already affected by, a disease or its complications, are asked a question or offered a test to identify those individuals who are more likely to be helped than harmed by further tests or treatment to reduce the risk of disease or its complications' (National Screening Committee, 2006). Assessment, on the other hand, provides an in-depth approach to establish a diagnosis and to identify management or treatment strategies. For example, a patient may have an oral health screening which may establish the presence of oral disease – perhaps plaque or painful gums – and assessment will establish whether this is a physical, psychological or social problem and nursing care can be established with the patient to treat or alleviate the problem(s).

Nursing diagnosis

The nursing diagnosis is made after the assessment stage on considering the patient's physical, psychological, spiritual or sociocultural reaction to their disease process or medical condition. The nursing process involves dealing with all aspects of a patient's care, including but beyond their original diagnosis. For example, a doctor may diagnose a patient with a chest infection and it will be up to the nurse to (know to) help the patient wash because the patient is too breathless to wash themselves. This is a new component of the nursing process.

This diagnosis of patient's problems then allows the nurse and the patient to prioritise the problems, which may be **actual** or **potential**.

Actual problems are those that exist at the time of assessment, for example breathlessness due to a chest infection. Potential problems are those that are at risk of developing if nursing interventions are either not implemented or are ineffective. For example, breathlessness may reduce the patient's ability to wash or remain continent, which in turn can lead to pressure sores. Therefore, although pressure sores are not present on admission, they may develop if nursing interventions are not put in place, or if the interventions are not effective.

An inability to meet personal hygiene needs may be an actual problem, but this inability can lead to several potential problems for the patient. If, for example, toenails are not cared for, the patient's mobility may be reduced; if dentures are ill-fitting, the patient may develop abrasions of the gums and reduce their nutritional intake. Both scenarios will in turn lead to an increased risk of pressure sores.

Planning stage

The nursing role is to prevent potential problems occurring and to solve or alleviate patients' actual problems. Once the patient's actual and potential problems have been identified, explained and discussed with the patient, the planning stage can commence. Planning involves discussing and identifying with the patient how these problems can be addressed in order to achieve the desired (by both the patient and nursing staff) outcome of nursing care. This involves establishing realistic goals (written statements of outcomes) which nursing interventions can help the patient achieve. Determining timescales for achievement of the goals is also important. For example, a patient may require education and help to achieve independence in meeting oral hygiene needs after a stroke. This may not be achievable in three days but may be achievable in two weeks. Often a series of small/short-term goals are required in order to achieve a longer-term overall goal. The plan of care is written to identify the nursing interventions, patient input and length of time required to achieve these goals. This care plan may be uni-disciplinary (i.e. a nursing care plan only) or multi-disciplinary (i.e. whereby all healthcare professionals contribute to the patient's plan of care).

Implementation stage

The implementation stage centres on carrying out the interventions identified in the care plan and monitoring the patient's reaction to them. This stage should support the medical input as well as the input of other professionals, for example the occupational therapist or the dietician. The core aspect of nursing interventions at this stage is to achieve the agreed goals and outcomes while alleviating illness and promoting health and, where possible, optimum independence.

Part of the nurse's role during this stage is to act as an educator and teach the patient. This may be about how to learn new ways of achieving hygiene after illness or trauma or to explain why aspects of maintaining hygiene may be important to the patient's overall health. For example, the patient may not realise the links between ill-fitting or broken dentures, poor nutritional status and delayed wound healing.

Therefore, for a nurse to be able to carry out interventions effectively with the patient's knowledge and cooperation, knowledge of theory and clinical procedures is vital.

Evaluation

Sometimes described as the final part of the nursing process, evaluation of the effectiveness of the implementation stage (and nursing interventions) allows the nurse and patient to monitor and judge whether the goals and outcomes have been achieved. However, the systematic approach is a continuous process and evaluation is a constant aspect of nursing care. Depending on the care situation and the health status of the patient, some care interventions will need to be evaluated on an hourly, and sometimes daily, weekly or even monthly, basis.

Patients in a high-dependency ward or intensive care may require their condition to be monitored hourly; patients in a residential home specialising in caring for older people may need some aspects of care, for example pain control, continuously monitored and oral health care monitored weekly or monthly.

Methods of evaluation are similar and use the same tools as initial assessment. The new data collection allows the nurse to identify if there are changes in the patient's condition and to determine whether the nursing care has been effective or whether the assessment phase must be repeated. Non-achievement of goals may be due to a variety of influences; the patient's overall physical condition may have deteriorated, for example through acquiring an infection; the data collected may not have provided all the information required; the interventions chosen to meet the goals may not have been the correct choice; or the goals may have been too ambitious and therefore unachievable.

The nurse will then have to reassess the patient and, using the data collected, proceed through the nursing process, changing the goals and/or nursing interventions if necessary.

Care planning

Nursing care plans are identified as essential in the delivery of modern nursing care (Björvell *et al.*, 2003), their purpose being a reflection of the patient's needs and wishes and a rationale for nursing interventions. Therefore, patient records should include transparent documentation which is completed in a manner that provides a basis not only for assessment and interventions but also for continuous evaluation and reassessment both of the patient's condition and the nursing interventions. Björvell *et al.* stress the role of nursing documentation in communication between colleagues and the patient and identify that individualised care plans strengthen the potential for patient participation in the decision-making process.

Owing to the diversity of patients and their conditions, it is unlikely that hygiene needs remain static. The patient may be recovering from illness and so becoming more independent or a crisis in health can result in dependency increasing, and so required interventions will naturally change. Ongoing reassessment of the patient's ability and needs is vital at least on a daily basis. Evaluation of care delivered in terms of the relationship of hygiene measures to other areas of care is also imperative, for example poor hygiene care may exacerbate skin problems and untreated urinary incontinence may increase the need for hygiene care.

ROPER, LOGAN AND TIERNEY MODEL FOR NURSING

The cyclical nature of the nursing process is demonstrated through the above descriptions of the stages. Using a framework for the nursing process guides the nurse. Using the Roper, Logan and Tierney (RLT) model for nursing contributes towards individualising patient care.

The current RLT model revised in 1996 (Roper *et al.*, 1996) is based on a model for living (Tomey, 1998). The main concepts of the model are that people are engaged in a process of living from conception until death and that, in order to live, 'activities of living' (ALs) must be carried out. The ability to manage these activities changes – possibly several times and to different degrees – throughout the lifespan. The model incorporates five concepts (Roper *et al.*, 1996; Holland, 2008). The five concepts are:

1. The 12 activities of living
2. The influence of lifespan (age)
3. The influence of the dependence–independence continuum
4. Factors influencing ALs
5. Individuality in nursing (normal living).

The 12 activities of living (Box 1.4)

- Represent the activities engaged in by all individuals whether sick or well.
- Are often seen as the main focus of the model but self-care abilities are influenced by the other four factors.
- The choice of ALs is influenced by Maslow's (1987) Hierarchy of Needs.

Box 1.4 Roper, Logan and Tierney's activities of living (ALs)

1. Maintaining a safe environment.
2. Breathing.
3. Communicating.
4. Mobilising.
5. Eating and drinking.
6. Eliminating.
7. Personal cleansing and dressing.
8. Maintaining body temperature.
9. Working and playing.
10. Sleeping.
11. Expressing sexuality.
12. Dying.

The influence of lifespan (age)

- Described by the stages of prenatal, infancy (0–23 months), childhood (2–12 years), adolescence (13–19 years), adulthood (20–64 years), older age (65+ years).
- Each stage is characterised by physical, intellectual, emotional and social developments.

The influence of the dependence–independence continuum

- Represented by a straight line.
- People move in either direction, depending on their circumstances.
- The goal of nursing is to enable the patient to acquire optimal (best) functioning in each activity (not necessarily independence, as this may not be a realistic goal).
- Assessment is needed to identify what the patient could/ could not do before and what were their previous coping strategies.

Factors influencing ALs

- Physical.
- Psychological.
- Sociocultural.
- Environmental.
- Politico-economic.

Individuality in nursing (normal living)

- How the person carries out the AL.
- How often is the AL carried out?
- Where is the AL carried out?
- Why is the AL required?
- What is known about the AL?
- What are the patient's beliefs about and attitudes towards the AL?

The RLT model has been criticised on the grounds that the concept of holistic nursing is not clearly defined in comparison to other nursing models. Nurses in particular are accused of not properly integrating the influencing factors but focusing instead on the care of the physical factors affecting these activities. Roper *et al.* (1996) argue that each AL is not as simple and straightforward as it looks; although some ALs have a biological basis to them, for example maintaining body temperature, others, such as those relating to personal dress, cleanliness, sexuality and the nature of work and play, have clear sociocultural influences.

Scenario 1.2

Ali is a 52-year-old gentleman who was admitted to the ward after being diagnosed as having had a stroke.

He has a right-sided weakness (hemiparesis) and has some problems with speaking, although he can understand what is being said. His wife visits daily, but they are both having difficulty coming to terms with what has happened to Ali.

On admission, Ali was assessed as having difficulty with balance, eating, washing and continence.

Using what you know about the nursing process and RLT model for nursing, think about how you would go about helping Ali and his wife to identify short-term goals to improve his condition. Consider whether you could involve other allied health professionals.

Suggestions for Scenario 1.2

You could carry out assessments of how dependent/independent Ali is in managing the skills. You may also decide to refer to allied health professionals – the physiotherapist, the speech and language therapist, the dietician and the occupational therapist – for specialist assessments. You may decide to use a nutrition screening tool for Ali and explain how it can monitor his progress.

You could discuss with Ali and his wife if he prefers what he thinks are the most important priorities to be addressed. You could use your theoretical knowledge to help Ali and his wife to understand why he has these problems and you could explain to Ali and his wife the potential problems that may occur if his current problems are not addressed.

You could explain the options for short-term goals, the skills involved and how Ali can contribute to his own care.

None of the ALs is independent. Problems in managing one AL will almost certainly affect at least one other AL. Nursing assessment requires the nurse to have the theoretical knowledge to be aware of the interlinking of each AL. Areas for general assessment of ALs relating to personal cleansing and dressing are noted below. Later chapters will identify any specific assessments that should be carried out in addition to the general assessment.

Maintaining a safe environment

- Is the patient able to understand risks and dangers?
- Does the patient pose any risks to other patients (e.g. the presence of infection)?
- Is the patient immunosuppressed?
- Is the patient pain free?
- Does the patient need a pain assessment?
- Is the patient's skin intact?
- What is the patient's pressure sore risk?
- What environmental factors in the clinical area or the home pose a risk to the patient?
- Does the patient have any allergies to prescribed treatments or medications?

Breathing

- Does the patient have an illness that affects breathing?
- What is the patient's rate of respiration?
- Is the patient breathless on exertion?
- Is the patient receiving oxygen therapy?
- Does the patient's breathing adversely affect their ability to self-care?
- Do breathing difficulties render the patient too anxious to meet hygiene needs?

Communicating

- Is the patient physically able to communicate their needs?
- Is the patient cognitively able to communicate their needs?

- What other influences may be preventing the patient from communicating their needs?
- Does the patient have problems with vision?
- Does the patient have problems with hearing?
- Can the patient understand what is being communicated?
- If not, what problems are influencing the patient's ability to communicate?

Mobilising

- Is the patient fully mobile?
- What physical problems does the patient have with mobility?
- Has admission to care affected mobility?
- What may be the cause of these problems?
- Does the patient have any psychological problems that may affect their mobility?
- Does the patient need a falls risk assessment?
- Are there any environmental problems that may contribute to mobility problems for the patient?

Eating and drinking

- What is the patient's nutritional risk?
- Are there any patient problems with eating and drinking that are affected by poor oral health?
- Are there any eating and drinking problems that will adversely affect the patient's personal cleansing/oral hygiene, e.g. is the patient nil by mouth?

Eliminating

- Does the patient have elimination problems, e.g. infection?
- Is the patient continent of urine?
- Is the patient continent of faeces?
- Does the patient use urinary continence aids?
- Does the patient use aids to faecal continence?

- What elimination problems will affect the patient's personal cleansing?

Maintaining body temperature

- What is the patient's temperature?
- Is the patient prone to feeling the cold?
- Is the patient pyrexial (have a high temperature)?
- Is the room a comfortable temperature?
- Is the patient able to adjust their clothing if they become too warm or too cold?

Working and playing

- Does any aspect of the patient's occupation pose a risk to maintaining personal hygiene, e.g. skin conditions?
- Do any of the patient's lifestyle choices impact on the patient's personal hygiene?

Sleeping

- Does the patient require any hygiene interventions overnight, which may disrupt sleep?
- Are there any personal hygiene problems which currently or may disrupt sleep?
- Does the patient require a special bed/mattress/linen?
- Does the process of carrying out personal hygiene interventions independently exhaust the patient?

Expressing sexuality

- What hygiene activities does the patient view as important in expressing their gender?
- What problems relating to personal hygiene may be causing difficulty with intimacy?
- What personal hygiene factors may impinge on the patient's ability to form relationships?
- Are there any hygiene problems that the patient perceives as preventing them from having an active sex life?

Dying

- What hygiene interventions are needed to improve the patient's comfort?
- What hygiene interventions may cause the patient discomfort?
- Does the patient require additional pain relief before any hygiene interventions?
- Do the relatives wish to participate in hygiene care?
- Are there any cultural/religious requirements relating to dying and personal hygiene?

THE CARE ENVIRONMENT IN RELATION TO PERSONAL CLEANSING

Maintaining a safe environment

In a follow-up to *Essence of Care* (Department of Health, 2001), the DH (2007) developed a further set of benchmarks to encourage best practice in achieving an optimum environment for care to be carried out in any care setting. The entire document has two main focuses. One area of attention relates to personalising the environment to suit patients' ages, culture, gender and allowing best access to individuals with varying abilities. The other main focus is on the safety of the care environment, with three factors against which local practice can be benchmarked (Table 1.3).

Aside from these benchmarking statements, to ensure the care environment is safe there are other general areas of assessment which are common to all patients, these are:

- Infection control.
- Moving and handling.
- Health and safety.
- Prescribed care.

Assessing infection control risks (patient)

One in 10 patients will develop a hospital-acquired infection (HAI). The costs of HAI are high to the patient through increased length of stay, increased fear and increased risk of death for some

Table 1.3 *Essence of Care* factors for the care environment

Factor No.	Factor title	Benchmark of best practice	Examples provided (relating to personal hygiene)
3	Well-maintained environment	People experience care in a tidy and well-maintained environment	There is no litter and bins are readily available The area is the appropriate temperature Toilet, bathroom and shower areas are free from clutter There is sufficient storage for patients' belongings Linen and laundry segregation; storage and disposal are well managed and appropriate Repairs are carried out promptly
4	Clean environment	People experience care in a consistently clean environment	Cleaning arrangements are flexible to meet the needs of the patients Regular routines for cleaning and managing of waste are in place that meet the national standard
5	Infection control precautions		Patients are informed why specific infection control measures are taken Staff wear personal protective equipment (PPE) as appropriate, changing between dirty and clean tasks and each episode of care Systems are in place to replace mattresses, mattress covers, baby changing mats, exercise mats, exercise mattresses, cushions, commodes and curtains, as appropriate

(*Source:* Department of Health, 2007)

patients and to the NHS through longer admissions, longer waiting lists, increased care costs and resource use.

Any general assessment of infection control risks for every aspect of personal hygiene includes the patient's current infection control status: does the patient have a current infection? Has the patient got a history of contracting infection(s)? Is the patient at particular risk of contracting infection? If the patient has an HAI, it is expected that healthcare staff follow a structured process in order to identify the root cause of how the infection was passed on to the patient and to learn from the process in order to prevent further spread (National Patient Safety Agency, 2007). Particular illnesses and infections which require monitoring and action to prevent the risk of spreading include (NHS Scotland, 2005):

- *Clostridium difficile*.
- Diarrhoea and vomiting or gastro-enteric infections.
- Influenza.
- MRSA (methicillin-resistant *Staphylococcus aureus*).
- Scabies and lice.
- Shingles (varicella zoster virus).
- Tuberculosis.

Poor infection control measures while carrying out hygiene procedures – in particular bathing, showering and oral hygiene – increase the risk of cross infection. Patients who will require particular assessment for both the presence of infection and the risk of infection include:

- Infants and people over 65 years.
- Patients with wounds of any kind, e.g. pressure sores or trauma.
- Patients admitted for surgery, i.e. pre- and post-operative patients.
- Patients who are immunosuppressed (have a lowered resistance to disease) through illness or medical treatment.
- Patients who undergo radiotherapy or chemotherapy.
- Patients who undergo invasive treatment (treatment that involves inserting medical equipment into the body which

may instigate an inflammatory response), e.g. intravenous infusions, urinary catheters, parenteral feeding tubes, wound drains.

Nursing staff will be required to assess what PPE is appropriate and when it must be used. It is important throughout this book to take note of whether procedures are clean or sterile/aseptic, as how and when gloves are worn will vary. Wearing a plastic apron means that the contact surface of the nurse's uniform is non-penetrable by water, blood or body fluids. This reduces the risk of transferring infection from patient to patient, patient to nurse or within different areas of the clinical environment (Dougherty & Lister, 2008).

The assessment of the patient will determine whether a patient is suitable for a bath or shower, or whether bed bathing would be the best option from a risk assessment perspective.

Assessing infection control risks (environment)

The thorough cleaning of bathrooms, shower rooms, toilets and all equipment used is vital to prevent cross-infection. Local policy should be used for general hygiene measures with specialist interventions used for patients who have known infections such as MRSA or *Clostridium difficile*.

To prevent cross-infection items such as toiletries, towel bales and specialist equipment (e.g. moving and handling equipment) should not be stored in bathrooms or toilet areas. Equally, all patients' personal toiletries and equipment should be used exclusively by the patient; disposable equipment should be used where possible, for example wipes. Single-use equipment should indeed only be used once before being sent for sterilisation.

Cleaning and effective decontamination and sterilisation (Table 1.4) of all reusable equipment such as dental examination equipment, hoists, baths and showers is integral to protecting the patient (NHS Executive, 2000). Each item should be cleaned on the basis of risk assessment for each patient who has used or will use the equipment.

Table 1.4 Cleaning, decontamination and sterilisation assessment of reusable equipment

Patient situation	Infection control measure	Level of infection risk
Equipment used for non-infected people with healthy, intact skin	Cleaning as per local policy	Low
Equipment which has had contact with bodily fluids After use with infected patients Before use with patients vulnerable to infection	Decontamination as per local policy	Medium
Equipment to be used with mucous membranes Items to be introduced with broken skin	Sterilisation	High

(*Source:* Damani, 1997)

Assessing moving and handling risks

Possibly up to 120 million days are lost from work through back injury (Health and Safety Executive, 2000). Many nurses in the past have admitted not using moving and handling equipment, even when it has been available (McGuire *et al.*, 1997) and nearly as many nurses have complained that what equipment is available is either not suitable or not in good working order (Moody *et al.*, 1996).

The bath/shower room is an area where patient and nurse safety may be compromised in many ways. Before planning how to best meet a person's hygiene needs a comprehensive moving and handling assessment must be carried out.

Often bath/shower rooms are small, restricting movement particularly if moving and handling equipment is required. In these circumstances healthcare staff, just as much as patients, are at risk of injury. Bath/shower rooms must be equipped with grab rails and handles that have been placed strategically where the patient can use them to facilitate safe standing/transferring. These may be wall-mounted, fixed to the floor or may be integral to the bath or shower. Occasionally, these aids can actually make mobility more difficult, for example floor-to-ceiling poles can stop equipment being taken right up to the bath or shower. It should be remembered that not all aids will be suitable for all people in all circumstances and that individual assessment remains vital (Swann, 2005).

Bath and shower seats are available for assisting patients to balance while washing. There are several variations; some may be discrete units which can be used for either the bath or the shower, some attach to the bath when needed and are equipped with harnesses for safety; others have inbuilt transfer systems. It should be remembered that people may have just as much difficulty getting out of the bath as getting in and this process can put severe strain on carers' musculoskeletal systems.

Assessment involves considering risks relating to equipment, processes and activities (e.g. using a patient hoist) that may cause harm (Rinds, 2007).

Core equipment identified for moving and handling should be available in every clinical setting (Table 1.5). Community-based patients should have had an assessment that identifies which equipment can be made available for use to assist the patient, carers and healthcare staff in the home. Equipment to assist moving and handling usually falls under one of three categories (Nazarko, 2005):

- Equipment to aid independence: for patients who have slightly reduced mobility but can weight bear and have both upper- and lower-body strength, e.g. grab rails.
- Equipment to assist with moving: requires nursing/carer intervention but patient retains some upper- and/or lower-body strength, e.g. standing hoist, turntable.
- Equipment to move the full weight of the person: requires at least two nurses as patient has very little or no upper/lower-body strength, e.g. tracking hoist.

Patients with special needs, for example those who are very overweight, may need specially ordered equipment (Rush, 2004). Specific assessment should also be carried out relating to any equipment used with the patient:

Table 1.5 Core moving and handling equipment required to carry out personal hygiene interventions

Type	Intervention	Rationale for use
Electric profiling beds	Bed bathing Transferring Ear, eye, nail and hair care; oral hygiene practices	Increases independence: patient can rise and change position using electronic buttons Reduces the load on the patient's sacrum The patient can vary the bed height independently; ease of transfer Reduces the risk of back injury for carers Modern beds can turn the patient in bed **NB:** Mattresses may not always be compatible with standard moving and handling equipment
Glide sheets/slide sheets	Bed bathing Transferring Sitting up in bed	Made of low-friction, lightweight materials which allows multidirectional glide Reduces shearing force Reduces friction **NB:** Cannot be used on a dynamic mattress unless the mattress is static
Manual transferring turntable	Transfers only – patient **must be able to weight bear**	Allows transfer from seating or lying equipment Can be used for patients who can stand but have difficulty walking/moving their lower limbs
Shower chair Transfer chair	Showering Accessing bath/shower room	Allows dignified transfer of patients (unlike wheelchairs the plastic is easily cleaned to prevent cross-infection) **NB:** These chairs should always be used instead of transferring using a commode (preserves dignity and privacy)
Mechanical standing hoists	Transferring from: • bed to chair (and back) • bed to commode or shower chair (and back) • chair to toilet (and back) • chair to seating (and back)	Allows patient to achieve a standing position while the upper body is supported by a sling Used for sit-to-stand and stand-to-sit transfers Allows the patient to have genitals and buttocks washed after using the toilet Allows changes of clothes after bathing **NB:** The patient must be able and willing to cooperate or they may fall through the sling onto the floor.

Table 1.5 *Continued*

Type	Intervention	Rationale for use
Patient hoists (full body sling hoists)	Facilitates any type of movement (raises patient from the bed; transfers patient) Bed making Transfer to shower chair Transfer to patient transfer chair	Used for patients who have little or no independent mobility Some are designed for use with immersion baths Some have weighing scales attached for monitoring the patient's weight **NB:** Patient must be able cooperate and understand the procedure; otherwise, their limbs may slip through the slings
Bath hoists	Allows patients to be transferred from transfer chair; raised on the hoist and lowered into an immersion bath	Movable arms allows the patient to access the hoist easily, e.g. using standing aid or turntable Used for patients who have sitting balance but poor lower-body strength **NB:** Does not have a smooth turning circle and cannot be used outwith the bathroom area Slings can be damaged by repeated water submersion and must be checked frequently for damage and weakness of the structure
Reclining/rising chairs	Helps a patient with limited mobility from a sitting to standing position	Assists with transfer to shower chair or bath hoist.
Adjustable-height baths	Raises the bath to a height suitable for nursing staff	

- Is the equipment in good working order?
- Is there a transparent checking and maintenance plan for the equipment?
- Have staff been trained in how to use and maintain the equipment?

- What is the impact of the equipment on the patient's dependence/independence?
- Is this the best equipment for the patient's situation and ability?
- How many nurses are required to carry out the procedure?
- Is the environment suitable for equipment use, e.g. is there enough room to manoeuvre the equipment?
- Is there a need to refer for specialist assessment, e.g. physiotherapy/occupational therapy?

One vital aspect of general assessment is to ensure that risk assessment forms trigger assessment of all aspects of the care processes (Rinds, 2007).

General health and safety

The risk of falls and injury can increase through hard surfaces becoming slippery if allowed to remain wet. Non-slip flooring is recommended but not always available; therefore, the use of non-slip mats and extra attention to keeping floors dry and free from spills such as water, soap or talcum powder is important. After each and every use, non-slip mats should be washed and dried according to local infection control policy and replaced frequently.

Obstacles in bathrooms and shower rooms can also pose difficulties for patients in terms of risk of falling (Hall, 2003).

Water temperature presents another potential hazard, particularly for some patient groups (Box 1.5). Patients have been scalded

---

Box 1.5 Patients who risk scalds and burns from hot water

- People aged 65+ years.
- Infants and young children, particularly newborn babies.
- People with learning disabilities.
- People who have epilepsy.
- People with poor mobility.
- People with circulatory or neurological disease.
- People with mental health problems.
- People with reduced cognitive ability.

---

and have even died after healthcare workers have failed to monitor the temperature of bathwater (Hill *et al.*, 2002). The DH (2002) recommends a water temperature of no more than 43°C for adults. Children under 18 months should not be exposed to water higher than 38°C (or lower than 36°C) (NHS Scotland, 2003), and until adulthood water temperature should not exceed 40°C (NHS Estates, 1998).

Bidets should be regulated to no more than 38°C and any water outlet that is not restricted to 43°C should be clearly labelled 'Very Hot Water'. Many baths and showers are currently available with inbuilt thermostatic control; however, the responsibility for patients' safety remains with healthcare staff, and water temperature should still be checked manually using a bath thermometer before being used by the patient. Nurses should be aware when patients use bathrooms and toilets that they may be at risk of burns or scalds from hot-water pipes, heated towel rails and radiators. Care must be taken to keep these covered safely (NHS Estates, 2007) and patients should be discouraged from leaning on these for balance.

Traditionally tepid (lukewarm) sponging has been recommended to lower temperatures of patients. The Royal College of Nursing (2008) cautions that using lukewarm sponging or baths with children risks actually raising their temperature as the practice may cause the blood vessels to constrict (become narrower), which will raise a temperature even further. The child may become so cold they shiver, which raises the metabolic rate and so raises their temperature. This is likely to be true of older people, who find it harder to maintain their temperature than younger adults do.

Patients who have cognitive problems, patients with learning disability and young children are at risk of accidentally ingesting personal toiletries such as brightly coloured shampoos or bath preparations. Cleaning fluids for infection control can also pose risks to these patients. Policies for the control of substances harmful to health (COSHH) should be followed (Health and Safety Executive, 2002) and patients should be advised about storing their personal toiletries safely.

Privacy and dignity are paramount to carrying out hygiene interventions, and intimate care must be carried out with sensitivity. Patients may feel the need to bath alone and lock doors, putting themselves at risk of help being delayed should they have an accident. A detailed and extensive risk assessment must be carried out which incorporates the expertise of the multi-disciplinary team and the wishes of the patient.

The decision as to whether patients can be supervised discreetly rather than accompanied in the bath or shower room depends on whether:

- The patient can get in/out of the bath/shower independently.
- The patient can sit up unaided and wash independently.
- The patient can make a safe decision regarding acceptable/comfortable water temperature.
- The patient's sensitivity to extremes of water temperature is not impaired.
- The patient has the mental ability to recognise dangerously hot water and take action.
- The patient is capable of calling for assistance if needed.
- The patient is able to exit from hot water independently.

Personal privacy may not be possible and patients will need to be encouraged to accept help with personal hygiene. This may be particularly relevant for children and teenagers who are self-conscious about their changing body and older patients who were raised during an era that was naturally more modest than current society.

PRESCRIBED CARE
What is prescribed care?

While many patients are able to meet their own hygiene needs or require minimal help to achieve the level of hygiene which satisfies their personal and social requirements, others will require hygiene interventions from a medical perspective. Nursing assessment contributes to this decision in that the patient may have identified problems with skin health, oral health, hearing or other deficits relating to personal hygiene which have occurred through a disease process.

Nurse prescribers

Resolving or alleviating these problems may require medical or specialist interventions. The patient is then likely to require medication or treatment under the category of prescription-only medicines (POM), which may only be prescribed by a qualified healthcare practitioner (e.g. doctor, dentist or qualified nurse prescriber). Nurse prescribers are registered nurses with an additional prescribing qualification recorded with the Nursing and Midwifery Council (2005). Like all registered nurses, independent/supplementary prescribers must work within their area of competence and will not be able to prescribe for children or people with mental health problems unless they are qualified to do so. Professional accountability demands that they prescribe only after a full assessment of the patient and only prescribe from the range of POM relating to their experience (Nursing and Midwifery Council, 2005).

Administering prescribed treatments

There are a range of POMs that could be prescribed for patients, but this book will mainly consider the range of topical prescriptions available. Oral medication (e.g. tablets, capsules) and injections are outwith the remit of this book. However, it must be emphasised that patients are likely to be prescribed medication under these categories. The registered nurse has an accountability to follow the standards for medication (Nursing and Midwifery Council, 2008) and to ensure that all staff are aware of possible side effects of medications which are being administered.

Unregistered nurses and prescribed care

Nursing students should not participate in medicine administration unless under supervision of a registered nurse and having been assessed as being competent to do so. The accountability rests with the registered nurse for deciding competence, but the responsibility lies with the nursing student to indicate if they feel any administration procedure is outwith their competence for stage of programme (Nursing and Midwifery Council, 2008). Unregistered nurses may have these duties delegated to them but, again, accountability remains with the registered nurse.

Patients who self-administer their medication

Many patients who are in care settings will be perfectly capable of administering their own medications. However, the responsibility for assessing capacity for self-administered medication (SAM) still lies with the registered nurse, and it must not be forgotten that a patient's condition can change dramatically and quickly.

Patients can be assessed for suitability to SAM at one of three levels:

Level 1

- The patient understands the POM being administered.
- The registered nurse must prompt the timing of the administration.
- The registered nurse must supervise the patient self-administering the medication.
- The registered nurse is responsible for the secure storage of the medicines.

Level 2

- The patient understands the POM being administered.
- The patient must prompt the timing of the administration and ask for the medication.
- The registered nurse must supervise the patient self-administering the medication.
- The registered nurse is responsible for the secure storage of the medicines.

Level 3

- The patient assumes responsibility for the full process including safe storage.

- The registered nurse has responsibility for continual assessment to ensure competence.

All levels must be recorded in the patients' documentation (Nursing and Midwifery Council, 2008). Parents and guardians of children in care can administer medication to their children under the same conditions. The British National Formulary (BNF) identifies a number of labels to be adhered to with different medications. It is important that all who may be administering prescribed care are made aware of any advisory labels (e.g. Label No. 28, 'To be spread thinly') and cautionary labels (e.g. Label No. 15, 'Caution flammable: keep away from fire or flames') issued with the medication (British National Formulary, 2008).

THE EFFECT OF AGE ON PRESCRIBED CARE
Infancy (0–23 months)

Newborn babies may be at risk of a reaction to any medication in the mother's breast milk. The amount of drug transferred in breast milk is rarely thought sufficient to obviously affect the infant. This applies particularly to drugs that are given parenterally (not using the digestive system). However, there is a theoretical possibility that the small amount of drug present in breast milk can induce a hypersensitivity reaction in the baby and so, if possible, medication should be avoided where possible (British National Formulary, 2008).

The risks to babies aged over 1 month is the same as for children. Babies less than 30 days old need particular care when prescribing and administering treatments. Babies of this age find it harder to clear drugs from their systems and risk toxicity (poisoning) from medication. This is particularly true of babies who are premature or jaundiced in the first few days/weeks of life (British National Formulary, 2008).

Childhood (2–12 years)

For safety reasons, children (like older adults and babies) are rarely included in drug trials, and so the presence of a licence does not necessarily indicate that a drug is suitable for a child or older person. Children therefore should always be prescribed medication with caution, and their age – and weight – should be taken into account and noted on any prescription documentation. It must be remembered that, although older children may have a weight similar to that of an adult, their organs do not have the same maturity and they may not be able to excrete the drugs from their bodies at adult doses. Dosages must be clearly prescribed in full to avoid accidental overdose.

A further consideration for children on long-term medication is the potential effect of medication, particularly liquids, on oral health. Sugar-free medication is preferable, or the child may be able to swallow solid doses and may prefer to do so (British National Formulary, 2008).

Adolescence (13–19 years)

There are few considerations for teenagers that are not also considerations for adults, although again teenagers are rarely included in drug trials.

Adulthood (20–64 years)

Adults and older adults have the greatest proportion of annual prescriptions. Many preparations may cause oral health problems even with short-term use. Antibiotics, for example, may cause oral thrush – a candidiasis-related fungal infection. Mouth ulcers can form as side effects from drugs, for example cytotoxic drugs (chemotherapy) and even non-steroidal analgesics; teeth can become stained even from some oral health preparations, for example some mouthwashes; the flow of saliva can be disrupted as a side effect of medicines such as antidepressants and analgesics (British National Formulary, 2008).

Pregnancy: medications can harm the embryo or foetus at any stage of the pregnancy not just the first trimester. When prescribing for a woman of childbearing age, and for men, assessment would include asking whether she was trying to conceive (British National Formulary, 2008). Many medications must be prescribed with caution and some topical preparations are included, for example steroid and antifungal preparations. Eye drops also require cautious prescribing as the medication (e.g. a steroid preparation) may be absorbed systemically.

Older people (65+ years)

Older people often have more than one disease occurring at the same time (multiple pathology), which may affect the number of medications they are prescribed. The more medications prescribed increases the risk of adverse drug interactions or reactions. The symptoms of these adverse incidents are sometimes confused by nurses as being part of normal ageing (e.g. reduced appetite, weakness, tiredness, confusion) and are not picked up on. However, normal ageing processes such as reduced liver and kidney function also mean that older people may have increased sensitivity to prescribed treatments (i.e. any allergies or reactions will appear faster and more severely than adults) and will not be able to secrete the waste from the drugs as efficiently as younger adults.

CONCLUSION

This chapter should have illustrated to the reader the importance of meeting personal hygiene needs for each patient. Assessment of every aspect of the patient's condition and the care environment is vital before, during and after carrying out nursing interventions. Nurses should refer to this chapter throughout the book for core assessment strategies.

REFERENCES

Ashurst A (2003) Maintaining client hygiene and appearance. *Nursing & Residential Care* **5**(3): 104–109.

Björvell C, Wredling R, Thorell-Ekstrand I (2003) Improving documentation using a nursing model. *Journal of Advanced Nursing* **43**(4): 402–410.

British National Formulary (2008) *British National Formulary*, 54th edn. Pharmaceuticals Press, London.

Damani N (1997) *Manual of Infection Control Procedures*. Oxford University Press, Oxford.

Department of Health (2000) *No Secrets: Guidance on developing and implementing multi-agency policies and procedures to protect vulnerable adults from abuse.* DH, London.

Department of Health (2001) *The Essence of Care: Patient-focused benchmarking for health care practitioners.* DH, London.

Department of Health (2002) *NHS Back in Work Campaign.* DH, London.

Department of Health (2007) *The Essence of Care: Benchmarks for the Care Environment.* DH, London.

Dougherty L, Lister SE (eds) (2008) *Royal Marsden Hospital Manual of Clinical Nursing Procedures*, 7th edn. Blackwell Publishing, Oxford.

Hall D (2003) Bathroom safety considerations for clients with a disability and their carers. *International Journal of Therapy & Rehabilitation* **10**(10): 473–475.

Hamilton P, Price T (2007) The nursing process, holistic assessment and baseline observations. In: C Brooker, A Waugh (eds), *Foundations of Nursing Practice: Fundamentals of holistic care* Elsevier, London, 349–389.

Health and Safety Executive (2000) *Musculoskeletal injuries from complex postures.* HSE, London.

Health and Safety Executive (2002) *The control of substances hazardous to health. Regulations 2002. Approved code of practice and guidance.* HSE Books, Sudbury.

Healthcare Commission (2007) *Spotlight on Complaints: A report on second-stage complaints about the NHS in England.* Healthcare Commission, London.

Hill A, Germa JF, Boyle JC (2002) Burns in older people: Outcomes and risk factors. *Journal of the American Geriatrics Society* **50**(11): 1912–1913.

Holland K (2008) *Applying the Roper–Logan–Tierney model in practice*, 2nd edn. Churchill Livingstone Elsevier, Edinburgh.

Horton R, Parker L (2002) *Informed Infection Control Practice*, 2nd edn. Churchill Livingstone, Edinburgh.

Kozier B, Erb G, Berman EJ, Snyder S (2008) *Fundamentals of Nursing: Concepts, process and practice.* Pearson Education, Harlow.

Maslow AH (1987) *Motivation and Personality*, 3rd edn. HarperCollins, New York.

McGuire T, Moody J, Hanson M (1997) Managers' attitudes towards mechanical aids. *Nursing Standard* **11**(31): 33–38.

Moody J, McGuire T, Hanson M *et al.* (1996) A study of nurses' attitudes towards mechanical aids. *Nursing Standard* **11**(4): 37–42.

Mousley M (2006) Diabetic foot screening: why is it not assessment? *Diabetic Foot* **9**(4), 192–196.

National Patient Safety Agency (2007) *Infection Control: Learning through action to reduce infection*. DH, London.

National Screening Committee (2006) *What is Screening?* NSC, London.

Nazarko L (2005) Safe moving and handling: A guide to hoists. *Nursing & Residential Care* 7(12): 551–553.

NHS Estates (1998) *Guidance Notes: 'Safe' hot water and surface temperature*. NHSE, London.

NHS Estates (2007) *Safe Bathing: Hot water and surface temperature policy*. NHSE, London.

NHS Executive (2000) *Health Service Circular 20001032: Decontamination of Medical Devices*. The Stationery Office, London.

NHS Scotland (2003) *Safe Hot Water and Thermostatic Mixing Valves (TMVs) Child Accident Prevention Trust, Bath Water Scalds Fact Sheet*. NHS Scotland, Edinburgh.

NHS Scotland (2005) *Infection Control Standards for Adult Care Homes: Final standards*. NHS Scotland, Edinburgh.

Nursing and Midwifery Council (2005) *NMC Standards: Standards of proficiency for nurse and midwife prescribers*. NMC, London.

Nursing and Midwifery Council (2008) *The NMC Code of Professional Conduct: Standards for conduct, performance and ethics*. NMC, London.

Pope AM, Snyder MA, Mood LH (1995) *Nursing Health and the Environment*. Committee on Enhancing Environmental Health Content in Nursing Practice, Institute of Medicine/National Academies Press, Washington.

Rinds G (2007) Moving and handling: Part two: Risk management. *Nursing & Residential Care* 9(7): 306–309.

Roper N, Logan W, Tierney A (1996) *The Elements of Nursing: A model for nursing based on a model for living*, 4th edn. Churchill Livingstone, London.

Royal College of Nursing (2008) *Caring for Children with Fever: RCN good practice guidance for nurses working with infants children and young people*. RCN, London.

Rush A (2004) An overview of equipment for moving and handling tasks. *Nursing & Residential Care* 6(5): 217–221.

Swann J (2005) Enabling residents to bath safely and easily. *Nursing & Residential Care* 7(9): 412–415.

Switzer J (2001) How to: Supervise a general bath. *Nursing & Residential Care* 3(5): 226–228.

Tomey AM (1998) The elements of nursing: A model for nursing based on a model of living. In: AM Tomey, MR Alligood (eds), *Nursing Theorists and Their Work*, 4th edn. Mosby, St Louis, 321–332.

Improving and Maintaining Oral Health | **2**

THE IMPORTANCE OF ORAL HYGIENE/HEALTH IN GENERAL PATIENT CARE

Oral disease is the most common disease the world over (Jones, 1998). Fifty to ninety per cent of the adult population in the UK and USA suffer from some form of gum problem (Coventry *et al.*, 2000). Plaque is visible in 72% of the UK population who have their own teeth; 43% of 15- to 18-year-olds have plaque and gingivitis (inflammation of the gums) (Harker & Morris, 2005).

Oral health overall has improved, although there are still patients in care settings with serious dental and oral problems. Mouth care may seem a fairly minor consideration when patients are acutely ill, but failing to maintain oral health can increase pain and infections. In terminally ill people, the health of the mouth is an indicator of quality of care (Denton, 1999).

The aim of this chapter is to help the reader understand the principles of carrying out mouth care and the underpinning rationale(s).

LEARNING OUTCOMES

After reading this chapter, the reader will be able to:

❑ Describe the anatomy of the mouth, tongue and teeth.
❑ Identify common diseases of the mouth during assessment.
❑ Discuss the rationale for using an oral health assessment tool.
❑ Carry out clinical care of the patient's mouth.
❑ Understand the evidence base underpinning clinical procedures.

DEFINITION OF ORAL HEALTH AND ORAL HYGIENE

Oral hygiene is often mistakenly thought to mean care of the teeth or dentures rather than all oral tissues and incorporates much more than merely the absence of disease (Gallagher, 1998).

Oral health is defined as 'a clean, functional and comfortable oral cavity; free from infection' and oral hygiene as 'the effective removal of plaque and debris to ensure the structures and tissues of the mouth are kept in a healthy condition' (Department of Health, 2001, p. 3).

THE ROLE OF ORAL CARE IN MAINTAINING GENERAL HEALTH

The pain and discomfort from chronic common oral problems affects a person's ability to function socially and psychologically. Discomfort causes loss of sleep, general irritation with family, friends and colleagues and increased sickness from work or education (Department of Health, 2005). If oral hygiene is not carried out, the normal flora of the mouth is disturbed by a build-up of bacteria over teeth and dentures. Plaque can form within 24 hours (Clarke, 1993). Dentures which are not cleaned properly can cause *candidiasis* (thrush), while bacteria in the form of plaque trapped under the dentures causes pain and inflammation of the mouth. This goes unnoticed if the inside of the mouth is not specifically examined (Frenkel, 2003). Plaque on natural teeth not only causes caries (cavities) and decay but inflammation of the gums (gingivitis). Chest infections can stem from uncleaned teeth or dentures (Fourrier *et al.*, 2000; Berry & Davidson, 2006) and in people who are unconscious and ventilated during acute illness (Joshipura, 2002). Oral hygiene is an area of care which is neglected in many clinical areas; up to 60% of patients may not be offered assistance with oral hygiene or have their dentures cleaned before sleeping for the night.

ANATOMY OF THE MOUTH (ORAL CAVITY)

The oral cavity (Figure 2.1) is lined with mucous membrane, which has a good blood flow and, providing there are no complications, heals relatively quickly if injured.

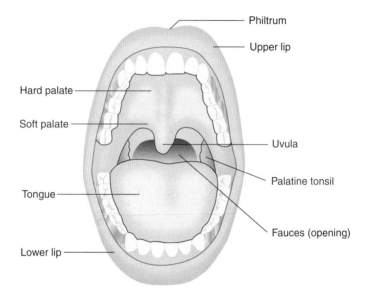

Figure 2.1 Structure of the oral cavity. From Thibodeau GA, Patton KT (2003) *Anatomy and Physiology*, 5th edn. Mosby Publishing. Copyright Elsevier. Reproduced with permission.

The roof of the mouth

The mouth can be divided into several areas. The **roof** (top) of the mouth is made up of the **hard palate** – the bony area towards the front of the mouth, which has little flexibility – and the **soft palate**, which is back nearer the throat and is mainly muscle tissue to help with swallowing.

The soft palate and the **uvula** (the soft structure hanging at the back of the mouth) prevent food and saliva from being accidentally ingested up into the nose.

The tongue

The floor of the mouth is made up of the tongue and its muscles, which function to make chewing and speaking possible. The

frenulum is the small membrane which can be seen attaching the underside of the tongue to the floor of the mouth.

The salivary glands

The mouth is lubricated by the secretions from three pairs of salivary glands. The wedge-shaped **parotid glands** are the biggest of the three pairs and are situated on each side of the jaw, just under and in front of each ear. The **submandibular glands**, which are around half the size of the parotid glands, secrete saliva at either side of the frenulum. The **sublingual glands**, which are the smallest glands, open into the floor of the mouth.

In addition to the three main pairs of glands, there are also around 600–1000 minor salivary glands, which are situated just under the mucosa lining the inside of the mouth, the nose, sinuses and the larynx (voice box). Saliva is required to lubricate and protect the lining of the mouth, allowing speech and eating without causing trauma through friction. The presence of saliva helps to bind food during mastication (chewing) to aid swallowing and provides the enzymes required to begin the digestive process (Jones, 1998).

The gingiva (gums)

The gingiva are the soft tissue which surround the roots of the teeth to keep them anchored in the mouth. Part of the gum is attached to the underlying bone and part forms the structure in which the teeth sit. Gum disease therefore increases the risk of tooth loss as the first part of the gum to be affected is the unattached margin.

ANATOMY OF THE TEETH

The teeth can be identified in three different parts (Figure 2.2).

The **crown** is the part that we see and is built to withstand constant use. Teeth are made up primarily of pulp – the nerves and blood vessels – surrounded by dentine, which makes up the bulk of the tooth, and are covered overall with enamel, which is the toughest tissue in the body.

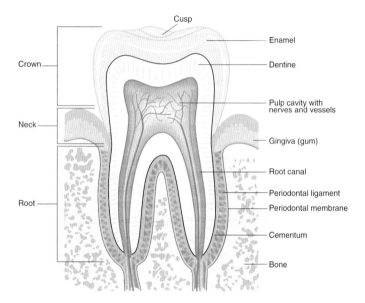

Figure 2.2 Anatomy of the tooth. From Thibodeau GA, Patton KT (2003) *Anatomy and Physiology*, 5th edn. Mosby Publishing. Copyright Elsevier. Reproduced with permission.

Teeth are formed differently according to their purpose: the front incisors are straight-edged for cutting and biting into food, the canine teeth at the side of the front teeth are pointed to tear food and the molars towards the back of the mouth are flatter on top to allow chewing.

The **neck** of the tooth is the narrower part at the bottom of the tooth and is engulfed by the gum. The third part of the tooth is the **root**, which sits in an individual socket in the jawbone. Each socket is lined with a periodontal membrane which holds the tooth to the bone. Each root is protected by a dental tissue called cementum, and has a canal through which the nerves and blood vessels pass.

Any disease in the enamel, dentin or cementum of the teeth will result in decay of the teeth known as dental caries or cavities in the teeth. The resulting holes in the teeth may expose the nerves and hence the pain caused by toothache. Disease or infection further down the tooth structure can cause gum abscesses or decay in the root of the tooth. This will then involve the dentist carrying out invasive root canal procedures to prevent the need to extract the tooth.

THE INFLUENCE OF AGE ON ORAL HEALTH (LIFESPAN)
Infancy (0–23 months)
Children's first teeth (which are known as their milk or baby teeth) develop before birth but only start to appear at around six months. The discomfort to babies during teething varies; symptoms include pain, excess salivation, facial flushing, inflammation of the gum and sleep disturbances (Chamley *et al.*, 2005). Other related symptoms may be individual to babies (e.g. an increased risk of nappy rash due to poor feeding). All 20 milk teeth should be through by the age of two. Some processed baby foods are very high in sugar and increase the risk of tooth decay (Ottley, 2002). It is important to begin toothbrushing with a small smear of toothpaste when the first teeth appear (British Dental Health Foundation, 2005). Dental advice can be sought regarding concerns about the use of fluoride toothpaste and toothbrush types.

Childhood (2–12 years)
Adult teeth begin to erupt around the age of seven. The molars are the last tooth type to grow in and this may take until the age of 21 years. However, the care of milk teeth is equally as important as second or adult teeth. The adult molars often appear before the first teeth have fallen out and there is a risk that these teeth will not be cared for effectively.

Dental caries are the most prevalent dental problem in children. The main cause is not the amount but the frequency of sugary food in the diet (British Dental Health Foundation, 2005).

Gum disease is rarely found unless due to disease, for example diabetes (Albino, 2002). Most children when in hospital do not require special mouth care unless they are being treated using radiotherapy, chemotherapy or are immunosuppressed. However, young children may not have the manual dexterity to brush their teeth effectively and therefore will require supervised mouth care at least until the age of seven years (British Dental Health Foundation, 2005). Mouthwash solutions should be used with care as younger children may not be able to swill their mouths and may swallow the liquid instead of spitting.

Adolescence (13–19 years)

Gum disease may start and if ignored increases the risk of tooth loss in earlier adulthood. Common problems may occur during the eruption of permanent teeth which may relate to the skeletal growth of surrounding structures. Dental and jaw disproportion is common in the UK (Scottish Executive Health Department, 2005). Young people may develop an over or under bite, where the upper and lower teeth are not aligned. Teeth may have gaps between them or may be crowded. By the age of 15, 35% of youngsters examined still had at least a moderate treatment requirement (Scottish Executive Health Department, 2005). Adolescence is often the age where the most effective corrections can be made as the teeth are still growing (British Dental Health Foundation, 2005). However, orthodontic interventions such as braces can cause embarrassment in teenagers and compliance with treatment can sometimes be problematic. Avoiding mouth infections from tooth jewellery or piercing is important. Teenagers may require education about the effects of smoking on oral health and how to maintain a healthy mouth through adulthood.

Adulthood (20–64 years)

The number of decayed, extracted and filled teeth continues to rise until about 35–40 years of age and then drops (Albino, 2000). Periodontal (gum) disease increases and presents as root caries. Adults have access to improved cosmetic dentistry, for example the use of veneers, tooth implants and whitening procedures. However, for those who do lose their teeth, there may be deeper psychological distress than during an era where tooth loss was more common. Oro-facial pain is a condition which affects many adults who are approaching middle age and older. In the absence of physical disease, such as arthritis, most instances of oro-facial pain are thought to reflect stress-related, learnt patterns of behaviour, such as tooth grinding or jaw clenching (Albino, 2000).

Older age (65+ years)

Older people are more likely to have tooth loss which adversely affects dental function; 75–95% of older patients are unable to eat properly (Zulkowski, 2003; Peltola *et al.*, 2005) and oral infections increase. Physical conditions affecting mobility and dexterity increase the incidence of oral and tooth disease. The more physically or cognitively disabled a person, the higher the risk of poor oral hygiene, denture plaque, oral disease and tooth or root decay (Simons *et al.*, 2001). Wearing dentures reduces chewing ability up to 40% compared to having enough teeth. Older people are more likely to be denture wearers and therefore are at risk of mouth ulcers, friction trauma from ill-fitting dentures and denture-induced stomatitis, including oral *candidiasis* (Fitzpatrick, 2000).

THE EFFECT OF DEPENDENCE IN ACHIEVING ORAL HEALTH AND HYGIENE

Oral care is seen as a low priority and there are nursing knowledge deficits in caring for many patient groups (Preston *et al.*, 2006; Ross & Crumpler, 2007; Southern, 2007).

There are some patient populations who may be at particular risk of oral health problems due to increased physical/cognitive dependency or an increased need for health education (Table 2.1). Patients who are unconscious or are dependent on carers should have the following oral hygiene measures as an alternative or in addition to normal hygiene measures discussed later in this chapter:

- Intubated patients should have their tubes repositioned and secured to avoid lip abrasions.
- Oral mucosa and tongue should be brushed or swabbed gently.

Table 2.1 People who may have an increased risk of poor oral health

Type of dependency	Relevant population
Physical dependency	People aged 65 years and over
	Children under the age of 8
	People with physical difficulties, e.g. stroke, Parkinson's disease, head injury
	People who are comatose
	Patients who have had any type of surgery
Cognitive dependency	People with a learning disability
	People with neurological conditions, e.g. dementia, head injury
	People with fluctuating consciousness levels, e.g. delirium
Requirement for health education	People undergoing chemotherapy and radiotherapy
	People prescribed medication affecting oral health, e.g. antibiotics
	People who have difficulty eating or who have a poor diet/are nil by mouth
	People who are prescribed oxygen therapy
	People who have type 1 or type 2 diabetes
	People who have iron-deficiency anaemia
	Women who are pregnant or have just given birth (hormonal changes can cause the gums to recede)
	People from socially deprived backgrounds

(*Source:* Roberts, 2000; White, 2000; Department of Health, 2005)

- Consider a saliva substitute to compensate for the drying effect of toothpaste.

PHYSICAL FACTORS INFLUENCING ORAL HEALTH

Patients with certain disease processes or trauma will have difficulty achieving their own oral hygiene needs and maintaining their own oral health. These range from patients who are intubated or fed nasogastrically to long-term chronic conditions which may impact on the patient's condition, for example they may be fed via percutaneous endoscopic gastrostomy (PEG). Scrupulous attention to oral health is needed as the patient will, in most instances, be nil by mouth (Griffiths *et al.*, 2000a). Patients who have joint and skeletal problems (e.g. arthritis), neurological disease (e.g. stroke, Parkinson's disease, nerve damage), respiratory or cardiac conditions and patients who have had oral or facial surgery will be at particular risk of being unable to maintain the dexterity needed to clean their teeth or to eat the types of foods (e.g. raw fruits and vegetables) which maintain oral health (NHS Quality in Scotland, 2005). Fatigue and/or pain due to ill health, acute or chronic, can reduce a person's ability and motivation to maintain their oral hygiene. The side effects of some prescribed treatments for physical conditions can cause added complications (e.g. dry mouth, dizziness and oral thrush).

PSYCHOLOGICAL FACTORS INFLUENCING ORAL HEALTH

Fear of the dentist is a significant barrier for a person's ability to maintain their oral health. However, people with mental health problems are likely to have poorer dental health than the general population overall. Occasionally, oral symptoms may be the first indicator of a mental health problem, for example people with anorexia bulimia may present with eroding tooth enamel, or burning mouth syndrome may be among the first physical indicators of anxiety or depression (Griffiths *et al.*, 2000b). People with mental health problems may lose the motivation, ability or understanding to benefit from oral healthcare. Medications prescribed for people with mental health problems can affect oral health, particularly from the side effects of dry mouth (xerostomia) (Griffiths *et al.*, 2000b). The long-term use of antipsychotic medications can result in tardive dyskinesias, which particularly affects movements of the mouth and tongue which can cause excoriation of the skin around the mouth as well as increasing difficulty for a carer to carry out effective mouth care (British Society for Disability and Oral Health/Royal College of Surgeons for England, 2001).

SOCIOCULTURAL FACTORS INFLUENCING ORAL HEALTH

Cost and fear are the most cited reasons for not accessing dental services. Certain population groups may be at particular risk of poor accessibility to dental care: homeless people, asylum seekers and groups who may encounter language barriers in accessing dental services (Griffiths *et al.*, 2000a; Department of Health, 2005). People from non-UK cultures may also be at increased risk of developing oral disease; those who smoke and drink alcohol increase their risk of developing gum disease and oral cancers. Chewing tobacco is a special problem among ethnic communities with their roots in Central, South and Southeast Asia particularly the older Bangladeshi community. Few people link the practice with mouth cancer and other serious diseases. However, few people also link diet and hereditary factors to the disease either (Scully & Bedi, 2000).

ENVIRONMENTAL FACTORS INFLUENCING ORAL HEALTH

There is evidence that some people, and particularly those with physical/cognitive dependence, are less able to attend dental care practices. The physical environment and architecture of many dental surgeries have been constructed in the past without consideration for disability, for example the situation of dental practices within tenement buildings (Oliver & Nunn, 1996). This inaccessibility of services results in personal costs of physical and emotional effort plus potential financial inequity (British Society for Disability and Oral Health/Royal College of Surgeons for England, 2001).

POLITICO-ECONOMIC FACTORS INFLUENCING ORAL HEALTH

NHS dental treatment costs are set annually by the Department of Health (DH) and are the same in each dental practice (Department of Health, 2001). However, the DH has initiated a review into the lack of access to NHS dental services within England and Wales (Smith, 2009). Few people use the NHS Direct helpline for information about accessing dental health care, and areas where there is a dedicated helpline for information have shown increased access to services (Croucher, 2003). Poverty and living in deprived areas is an indicator of poor oral health risk; poor health education and lack of money can result in choices of food and lifestyle which can lead to dental decay, oral cancers and the detrimental impact of medication on oral health (Department of Health, 2009).

ASSESSING ORAL HEALTH AND HYGIENE

An oral assessment consists of an inspection of the mouth to ascertain the oral health status of the individual (British Society for Disability and Oral Health/Royal College of Surgeons for England, 2001). All patients should have an initial simple screening of the oral cavity, in partnership with the patient's carers if necessary. It is particularly important that carers' views be sought when the patient is unable to communicate or cooperate with an oral health assessment (Chalmers & Pearson, 2005). However, while screening will identify the risk of developing oral health problems, comprehensive assessment is required for all those found to be at risk.

There are a variety of oral health assessment tools which are reliable and validated, which means that they have been tested on specific populations, for example patients in intensive care units or patients undergoing chemotherapy. However, each patient group has particular needs and risks to oral health and not every assessment tool will be valid. Care must be taken that the appropriate tool is used.

Oral health assessment involves both verbal and physical examination. The patient should be sitting comfortably and there should be adequate lighting (Dougherty & Lister, 2008). Assessing for individual patient needs depends on a set of principles that are interrelated (Table 2.2).

While carrying out assessment, nurses should always remember that many aspects of poor oral health are modifiable (i.e. can be improved) (Table 2.3).

Before careful physical examination of the mouth and oral cavity, take a written history of the patient/carer's perception of any oral problems and the impact these problems are having on the patient's well-being.

Table 2.2 Principles for assessing oral health needs

Principle for need	Influences on principles
Physical ability to meet own hygiene needs	consciousness levels specific disease process stage of recovery post surgery terminal illness
Psychological ability to meet own hygiene needs	cognitive status presence of disease delirium terminal illness fluctuating consciousness motivation presence of pain
Cultural care required to assist hygiene needs	specific beliefs around hygiene rituals
Safety requirements	coping ability patient's understanding of safety measures
Maintaining normal living	patient preferences for normal routine preferences for oral hygiene equipment
Infection control issues	following infection control procedures within clinical areas patient's personal equipment
Prescribed care	influenced by the need for medication, e.g. systemic drugs or topical treatment for oral conditions
Privacy and dignity	preserving patient autonomy through choice and involvement in decision-making and care planning

Procedure: Assessing oral health
Equipment

- Seat/stool × 2.
- Pen torch.
- Tongue depressor.
- Glass/tumbler/cup of cool water (if not nil by mouth).
- Receptacle for the patient to spit into.
- Suction equipment if required.
- Personal protective equipment (PPE): gloves and apron.
- Protective cover for the patient.
- Tissues or wipes.
- Gauze swabs.

Table 2.3 Assessment of oral health with modifiable interventions

Category	Assessment	Modifiable intervention
Voice	Speak to the patient and listen:	
Score 1	The voice is normal	Maintain usual routines
2	The voice has changed and is deep, hoarse or raspy	Refer to medical staff
3	Patient has difficulty talking or experiences pain	Refer to medical professionals and/or speech and language therapist
Swallow reflex	Ask patient to swallow and observe:	
Score 1	Normal swallow	Maintain normal routines
2	Pain on swallowing	Refer to medical staff
3	No swallow reflex/unable to swallow	Give assistance with oral hygiene; refer to speech and language therapist
Lips	Observation:	
Score 1	Smooth, pink, moist	Maintain normal routines; ensure adequate hydration
2	Dry or cracked	Apply water-based lubricant
3	Ulcerated, bleeding or inflamed	Refer to medical staff for prescribed interventions
Tongue	Observation:	
Score 1	Pink, moist and papillae present	Maintain oral hydration and normal oral hygiene routines
2	Coated or loss of papillae; shiny and/or redness	Clean with soft toothbrush and mild toothpaste; increase fluids, particularly water
3	Blistered; cracked; inflamed	Refer to specialist; document progress and prescribed interventions
Saliva	Using a spatula observe the centre of the tongue and the floor of the mouth:	
Score 1	The saliva is watery	Maintain normal routines
2	The saliva is thick	Increase fluid intake; offer iced water; offer alcohol-free mouthwash
3	No saliva	Refer to specialist for saliva substitute

Table 2.3 *Continued*

Category	Assessment	Modifiable intervention
Mucous membrane	Observe the mucous membrane in the oral cavity:	
Score 1	Pink and moist	Maintain normal routines
2	Reddened or coated; white but not ulcerated	Refer for prescribed care
3	Ulcerated with/without bleeding	Refer for prescribed care
Gingiva (gums)	Press gums (gently)with end of a spatula and observe:	
Score 1	Gums are pink and stippled and firm	Maintain normal oral hygiene measures
2	Gums are swollen with/without redness	Continue with brushing teeth but refer to specialists for prescribed care
3	Gums are bleeding with/ without pressure	Urgent referral to dental professionals
Teeth (if present)	Observe appearance:	
Score 1	Teeth are clean with no debris present	Maintain usual teeth-cleaning regime
2	Plaque or debris present in localised area (including between teeth)	Supervise oral care; refer for specialist cleaning
3	Plaque or debris present along gum/tooth line	Refer to dental professionals
Denture bearing area	Observe appearance:	
Score 1	Area is clean with no debris	Maintain usual denture hygiene measures
2	Plaque or debris present in localised area where dentures would be placed	Supervise oral hygiene care; ensure dentures are cleaned and rinsed after meals
3	Plaque or debris present along the line of the denture-bearing area	Refer to dental professionals; ensure teeth are removed overnight; continue with hygiene measures to the mouth

(*Source:* White, 2000; Singapore Ministry of Health, 2004)

Action	Rationale
Explain each step of any procedure or examination to the patient and gain their consent	Ensures the patient understands the process and encourages their cooperation
Ensure the patient is comfortable and can sustain the oral examination. Ask for a verbal response (if possible). Assess the patient's voice	Normal conversation reduces the patient's self-awareness and produces a more normal voice for assessment
Sit the patient in a good light source but avoid direct light(s) shining into the patient's eyes	
Ask the patient to rinse their mouth with the cool water and spit the residue into a receptacle	Clears the mouth of any easily removed debris before examination. Allows the nurse to assess whether the patient has normal mouth movements. e.g. no paralysis
Ask the patient to sip and swallow a small amount of cool water	Allows a swallow assessment. Allows rudimentary assessment of the patient's ability to coordinate eating, drinking and dexterity
Observe the patient's lips and surrounding tissue	Identifies any dryness, trauma or cracking of lips. Identifies the presence of chronic infection in the corner(s) of the mouth
Either sitting on a stool opposite the patient or standing behind the patient, ask the patient to open their mouth and stick out their tongue	Allows the nurse to assess the appearance of the tongue and to assess whether the patient has normal function (e.g. can the patient poke their tongue out symmetrically/normally?)
Using a pen torch and tongue depressor, inspect the inside of the mouth to assess the appearance of the saliva over the oral mucosa, the tongue and the floor of the mouth. **NB:** Ensure that the patient can tolerate the tongue depressor without gagging.	Using a pen torch maximises a light source and a tongue depressor keeps the tongue still enough for close examination of the oral cavity

Continued

Action	Rationale
Score the appearance of the saliva	
If the patient is unable to tolerate the tongue depressor, gently wrap a gauze swab round the tongue and move it manually. **NB:** Do not attempt this with patients who are unable to understand or cooperate	Performs the same purpose as a tongue depressor but may reduce gagging as the nurse has more hand control than with the depressor.
	The nurse must risk assess against the risk of being bitten by the patient
Using the tongue depressor and pen torch, assess the appearance of the oral mucosa	
Removing the patient's dentures (see below) if appropriate, gently prod the gums with the tongue depressor and assess the appearance of the gums	Assesses gum health and for the presence of gingivitis (gum disease)
If teeth are absent and/or the patient wears dentures or a bridge, check the gums for signs of debris where the dentures would normally sit	Assesses the hidden risks of oral health for denture wearers
If teeth are present, assess the teeth for obvious signs of decay, plaque or debris	Assesses the general health of the teeth and the presence of potentially debilitating tooth decay
Remove gloves and dispose of them and any used equipment into a clinical waste bag	
Giving the patient their oral hygiene equipment, ask them to carry out their own oral hygiene	Assesses whether the patient has the balance, ability, understanding and dexterity in carrying out the skills
Assess the patient's ability to access and use the equipment to self-care	
Return the patient to their chair/bedside and ensure that they are comfortable	
Identify from the assessment which problems require multi-disciplinary referral and which problems will respond to nursing interventions	Allows nursing diagnosis from the nursing assessment
Develop a nursing care plan with the patient to meet their goals for oral hygiene and health	Individualises nursing care
Document the screening score. Identify referrals and plan care with the patient, including evaluation periods	

Frenkel (2003) suggests that many nurses may be unaware of whether their patients have full or partial sets of teeth and are unaware of whether these patients are able to meet their own self-care needs for oral hygiene. Despite literature providing evidence for carrying out mouth care, many nurses and carers remain ignorant of how to carry it out effectively.

Oral hygiene equipment

To solve nursing problems relating to oral health and hygiene, a number of options are available to nurses.

Toothbrushes

Normal adult size toothbrushes may be difficult to handle and clean teeth effectively (Berry & Davidson, 2006), particularly for intubated patients, people with learning disabilities and anybody who has had oral/facial surgery. Larger toothbrushes are rarely effective in reaching the furthest aspects of the patient's mouth. While there is a substantial benefit in using toothbrushes over foam swabs for the removal of dental plaque (Pearson, 1996), standard hospital issue adult toothbrushes may be too hard-bristled to be tolerated by patients.

Soft toothbrushes

Bowsher *et al.* (1999) and the British Society for Disability and Oral Health/Royal College of Surgeons for England (2001) advocate the use of a soft toothbrush, despite it not being the nurse's first choice of oral hygiene tool. For all people with their own teeth and for care of dentures, using a soft-bristled 'baby' toothbrush provides improved access to all areas of the mouth and can also be used to gently brush the tongue. They are also effective in cleaning the gums of patients who wear dentures.

Children should always be given a child size toothbrush to use. While there is an acknowledged greater risk of soft tissue injury if used carelessly, using a toothbrush is more effective in removing food debris and plaque than foam sticks.

Power toothbrushes
Powered toothbrushes, which rotate in one direction and then the other, remove more plaque than manual toothbrushes and protect against gum inflammation (Robinson *et al.*, 2005; Sharma *et al.*, 2005). There is no more risk of injury than from manual toothbrushes and for many patients with dexterity problems they increase the effectiveness of tooth brushing.

Foam sticks/foam and cotton sticks
Foam sticks are popular with nursing staff. While there is less risk of trauma, particularly after oral surgery or in conditions which cause bleeding or clotting problems (Hahn & Jones, 2000), they have been found to be less effective in reducing plaque (Rawlins, 2001). They may be more effective if soaked in chlorhexidine mouthwash solution (Ransier *et al.*, 1995). Some clinical areas have removed them from use due to risk of certain patients biting off the foam and choking.

Lemon and glycerine swabs
Lemon is highly acidic, resulting in the teeth being stripped of calcium; glycerine draws moisture from the tissues. This interferes with effective saliva production, causing a dry mouth. There may also be an associated risk of damage to the tooth enamel with the citric acids and hypersensitivity of the oral mucosa in denture wearers (Milligan *et al.*, 2001). The acidic nature of glycerine and lemon swabs lowers the natural pH of the mouth and allows bacteria to flourish.

Interdental cleaners
The use of dental floss, and less commonly wood sticks (or dental swords), is often recommended by dentists and dental hygienists for more efficient plaque and tartar removal than toothbrushing alone or even the use of mouthwashes. If the patient is unable to use floss independently, flossing swords can be used as they are rigid (Denton, 1999). Careless use may cause gum injuries and problems; children should not use these for this reason and nurses should exercise extreme caution. It is important that

nursing staff are shown how to use the floss correctly, to mini-mise gum trauma. The floss is pulled tightly between two hands and manoeuvred between the teeth in a gentle seesaw action, up and down from the crown (top) of the tooth down towards the gum and along the gum line (Dougherty & Lister, 2008). A clean section of floss should be used for each tooth.

Cleaning equipment
Toothpaste
Toothpastes are the most widely used oral cleaning product; although it is not significant in plaque removal, certain types are useful in the prevention of tooth decay. Toothpastes range from decay/plaque-reduction formulae to specialist pastes for smokers, sensitive teeth and flavoured children's toothpaste. More recently, tooth-whitening pastes are becoming the most popular pastes used. To improve patient comfort and reduce halitosis (bad breath), the use of non-foaming toothpaste is preferable as it is more easily rinsed away, reducing the drying effect of residual toothpaste on the oral mucosa. Fluoride is the most effective cleansing agent (Department of Health, 2005). Whatever type of toothpaste chosen, the action on tooth cleansing will be more effective if the patient is encouraged to brush for three minutes and spit out the residue (British National Formulary, 2009).

Water-soluble v. paraffin- or glycerol-based products for lip care
Using water-soluble lubricating gels (e.g. KY Jelly) prevents the potential dehydration effects of glycerol or petroleum jelly on the lips. Petroleum jelly also leaves a sticky residue on the lips, which can cause discomfort for the patient and can attract additional debris. Patients themselves report that the use of unperfumed moisturising cream is the most acceptable treatment (Feber, 1995), but KY Jelly is also effective and easily absorbed.

The use of mouthwashes
Rinsing the mouth as part of basic hygiene requires a solution that will be both effective and pleasant to taste for the patient.

There are many choices for professionals to advise their patients to use. However, not all mouth solutions are suitable in all cases.

0.9% saline (normal saline)
This solution is almost tasteless, does not irritate the oral mucosa or change the salivary pH while promoting healing (British National Formulary, 2009).

Sodium bicarbonate
This is as effective as saline for removing debris but tastes less pleasant. The correct concentration must be used to prevent trauma/burning of the mucosa and increased bacteria levels from an alkaline mouth (Miller & Kearney, 2001).

Hydrogen peroxide
Removes bacteria and debris, but changes to the flora (normal bacteria) of the mouth can increase the risk of tissue damage if the mouth is ulcerated. Oral thrush can be an unwanted side effect.

Chlorhexidine mouthwash
The use of a chlorhexidine mouthwash after brushing the teeth reduces plaque and bacteria and improves gum health. The mouthwash has antibacterial, antifungal and anti-plaque properties (Sharma *et al.*, 2003) and therefore reduces the risk of colonisation of *Candida albicans*, which leads to oral candidiasis. However, the alcohol content can cause some patients severe discomfort and can have a drying effect on the mouth, and use should be restricted to twice daily. Chlorhexidine rinse is recommended for people who have acute gum problems. Long-term use, more than 3–4 weeks, is not generally advisable, as the teeth can be stained brown. There is less risk of this if teeth are cleaned first.

General (over-the-counter) mouthwashes
Many commercial mouthwashes are fairly effective in controlling plaque and gum disease but not as effectively as chlorhexidine.

There are also concerns about the amount of alcohol in some preparations. Some preparations also leave a dry mouth as a side effect and the alcohol content can increase any oral pain present (Milligan *et al.*, 2001).

PRESCRIBED CARE

Some patients may require prescribed preparations to address more complex oral problems such as a painful throat or a candidiasis yeast infection. Using any preparation, it is important to follow the advisory label provided by the pharmacy.

If a prescribed mouthwash solution is used, the patient should be encouraged to rinse the mouth for one minute and then spit it out (British National Formulary, 2009). Caution should be used with patients who may not have the understanding or physical ability to avoid swallowing the solution. It is advisable after any oral health intervention that the patient does not eat or drink for at least 30 minutes after use.

Artificial saliva

Artificial saliva is similar to the composition of natural saliva but does not have the same oral cleansing and protection effects. The preparations come in different varieties: mouth sprays (to replace saliva), lozenges or pastilles (to stimulate saliva production) or tablets (for salivary gland impairment) (British National Formulary, 2009). Alternative palliative nursing interventions can include offering the patient slivers of ice to suck, frequent sips of cool water or sugar-free lozenges/chewing gum. The patient must be carefully assessed for intact swallow before any of these interventions is used.

AIDS FOR ORAL HYGIENE
Mouth props

Mouth props literally prop the mouth open and can be used to assist the nurse carrying out mouth care procedures, particularly for paediatric, unconscious or sedated patients. They come in wedge shapes with grooves for the teeth or as scissor-type ratchets where the amount the mouth is opened is controllable. If no props are available in the clinical area, a makeshift prop can be made from winding gauze swabs over several tongue depressors and securing safely.

Modified toothbrushes
Toothbrushes can be accessed with modified candles to improve independence. They may be wide-handled, have added grip aids, Velcro straps or foam grips.

Floss brushes
Brushes which are supplied with dental floss are useful for patients with poor dexterity. Electric or powered floss brushes are even easier to use.

INFECTION CONTROL
Gloves should always be worn when carrying out oral care as protection for the patient and the nurse. Infection control principles should be adhered to for oral hygiene equipment, such as drying tooth care equipment thoroughly, and should not be stored in toilet bags or other containers. Toothbrushes should be renewed every 12 weeks (Jones, 1998).

COMMON ORAL HEALTH CONDITIONS
Halitosis (foul-smelling breath)
Some malodour on the breath is normal on waking and can be caused by spicy foods, smoking and alcohol (Department of Health, 2005). However, poor oral hygiene causes more serious malodorous breath, which is made worse by any form of infection in the mouth. Other causes can be traced to tooth decay, lack of saliva and pathologies such as tumours (Coventry *et al.*, 2000). Certain medications may cause bad breath and the symptoms of some diseases present with bad breath, for example ketoacidosis with unstable diabetes or renal and hepatic failure including cirrhosis of the liver.

People with halitosis may not be aware of the condition until they are told by another person. Once aware, people are often

> **Box 2.1 Interventions for treating/improving halitosis**
>
> - Improving the patient's oral hygiene by providing assistance as required and ensuring oral hygiene is offered as often as required on assessment.
> - Encouraging the patient to eat regularly, accompanied by fluids.
> - Offering additional hygiene measures after foods that can cause bad breath.
> - Encouraging the patient to chew sugar-free gum regularly but only after risk assessment for choking has been carried out.
> - Offering one of the many oral deodorants (breath fresheners) available over the counter. This may have to be approved by medical staff, dental staff or nurse prescribers to ensure that there are no contraindications to their use.
> - Using an antibacterial mouthwash, providing there are no contraindications to its use. Alcohol-based mouthwashes may not be suitable for all patients.
> - Providing the patient with toothbrushes which have tongue cleaners. (These are becoming more commonly available over the counter.)
>
> (*Source:* British Dental Health Foundation, 2005)

distressed and self-conscious. Halitosis can be reduced by referral to dental professionals for remedial oral treatment, including antibiotic therapy such as metronidazole, 200 mg three times daily for seven days. Nursing staff can prevent the onset or reduce the symptoms of halitosis by implementing the nursing interventions in Box 2.1.

Excessive saliva production

Some people, and particularly older adults; those with learning disabilities and people with neurological conditions experience excessive saliva flow, which can be embarrassing as well as difficult to manage. Constant saliva flow also can cause painful skin in the surrounding areas, such as the chin and neck. Swallowing problems and problems with poor muscle control can result in pooling of saliva in the mouth, leading to dribbling/drooling. Pharmaceuticals can reduce saliva flow but many of the side effects of these medications can outweigh the benefits. Nursing interventions can reduce the effects of excessive saliva production (Box 2.2).

Box 2.2 Interventions to minimise the effects of excessive saliva production

- Remind the person to swallow as much as is possible.
- Encourage the person to maintain as upright a position as is possible. Additional support and/or special seating may be needed.
- Prompt the person to keep their mouth closed.
- Encourage the person to flex their head forward when swallowing.
- Referral to the speech and language therapist may be of benefit to improve swallow ability.
- Barrier cream can be applied to the chin and neck to prevent excoriation from drooling that has been difficult to control.

Xerostomia (dry mouth)

Xerostomia is caused by a reduction or an interruption in the flow of saliva. A dry mouth causes discomfort and can interfere with speech and eating. Lack of saliva increases the risk of dental caries, gum disease and infections, as the mouth loses the natural protective and cleansing effect of saliva. The most common cause of dry mouth (aside from the normal effects of dehydration) is medication side effects, for example antihypertensives, sedatives and antidepressants (British National Formulary, 2009). Other patient groups at risk of dry mouth include:

- Patients undergoing oxygen therapy: causes drying of the oral and/or nasal cavities.
- Patients having radiotherapy to the head and neck areas may find that saliva production is reduced or halted completely for a significant period during and after treatment.
- Patients who have had extensive surgery: the side effects of the anaesthetic causes dry mouth by reducing secretion of saliva.
- Patients who are nil by mouth: oral hygiene is at risk of being neglected; dehydration is a risk.
- Patients undergoing radiotherapy for head and neck cancer: saliva gland function becomes impaired, sometimes irreversibly.

> **Box 2.3 Possible nursing interventions for management of reduced saliva**
>
> - Administration of saliva substitutes as prescribed. Although it should be remembered that these may not have a 'normal' taste for the patient.
> - Administration of mouthwashes as prescribed.
> - Encourage fluids as tolerated by the patient but avoid sugar-laden drinks if possible (lack of saliva reduces the natural cleansing effect).
> - Ensure that the patient is referred to dental services for assessment and remedial treatment if required.
>
> (*Source:* Fiske *et al.*, 2000)

It is important that nursing staff are aware of the impact of disease and the side effects of treatments and take action accordingly to reduce discomfort and the risk of further deterioration of oral health (Box 2.3).

Oral candidiasis (oral thrush)

This is an opportunistic oral infection caused by an overgrowth of *Candida spp* (yeast) that causes difficulty in eating and leads to an increase in systemic infections (e.g. chest infections). *Candida spp* commonly colonises the mouths of people who are immuno-suppressed, including people undergoing chemotherapy, people who are HIV positive, dependent older adults and people with systemic infection. Any candidal infection must be treated immediately with an antifungal agent and the mouth kept moist.

Cold sores

Many infants and young children suffer from primary herpes virus infection of the lips and oral mucosa. Many of these infections are subclinical (i.e. symptomless) but the viral presence results in the child developing future immunity. However, the virus can remain dormant in the lips and in adolescence and adulthood can recur. The cold sore begins with a nippy sensation on the area, which develops into a blister and then ulcerates. The cold sore usually lasts untreated for around two weeks.

Causes of cold sores

- Idiopathic: spontaneous recurrence with no obvious cause.
- Trauma, e.g. cut lips.
- Sunlight/sunburn.
- Hormone imbalance, e.g. menstruation.
- Stress.

The herpes simplex virus is highly contagious and any patient with a cold sore should have scrupulous hygiene measures and, where possible, not share washing facilities with other patients who may be vulnerable in contracting the virus. Nursing staff can advise patients to use sunscreens at all times to reduce the risk of developing sores. Acyclovir 5% is an antiviral preparation that should be used at the onset of the tingling feeling, which signifies the development of a cold sore (British National Formulary, 2009). Patients should be warned to expect itching or drying of the skin as a side effect.

Gingivitis

This condition is characterised by inflammation of the gingiva (gums) and is caused mainly by ineffective oral hygiene, which allows bacterial plaque formation between the gums and the teeth (Berry & Davidson, 2006). Studies in the USA and the UK suggest that *some* degree of gingivitis affects 50–90% of the adult population (Coventry *et al.*, 2000).

Signs and symptoms

- Gums will bleed with tooth brushing, flossing or gentle probing.
- Gums show swelling and redness along the base of the tooth/teeth.
- The gums may change shape e.g. thickened and bulge.
- Pain may be present.

Risk factors

- Ineffective hygiene measures.
- Smoking.
- Increasing age.
- Diabetes.
- Pregnancy.
- Reduced immunity, e.g. those undergoing chemotherapy.
- Intubation.

Initial referral is required to a dental professional for full cleaning and scaling of the teeth for plaque removal. Gingivitis can be reversible if treated with antibiotics and oral hygiene is continued (Dougherty & Lister, 2008). Occasionally, people may be under the misapprehension that the cause of bleeding is the actual brushing and may stop oral hygiene. This is not the case, and gentle brushing should be encouraged. However, advice could be offered about using a soft toothbrush with a small head.

Periodontal disease

Periodontal disease occurs when gingivitis has been ineffectively treated (Figure 2.3). The inflammation spreads below the gum level involving the bone and the periodontal membrane, which anchors the teeth to the bone. The risk factors are the same as for gingivitis, but continuing inflammation results in separation of the gum from the tooth (Sharma *et al.*, 2003). The periodontal ligament breaks down and the adjacent alveolar bone is destroyed. At this stage of periodontal disease, the teeth will begin to loosen and will eventually fall out.

The symptoms are similar to gingivitis but may also include:

- Halitosis.
- Foul taste in the mouth.
- Recession and associated root sensitivity.
- Drifting/loosening of teeth, causing difficulty in eating.
- Periodontal abscess (which may cause pain).

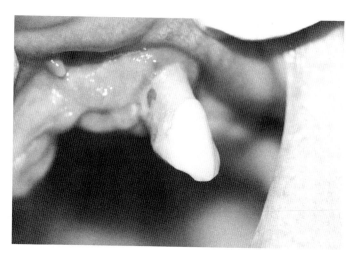

Figure 2.3 Periodontal disease. From Hollins C (2008) *Basic Guide to Dental Procedures.* Reproduced with permission from Wiley-Blackwell.

Unlike gingivitis, periodontal disease is usually irreversible and so prevention of periodontal disease is therefore vital. Advice to patients should include brushing the teeth at least twice daily with, if possible, a powered toothbrush. If the patient has a problem using a toothbrush, dental advice must be sought. Flossing or using interdental sticks on the teeth at least three times a week is advisable and people with predisposing factors should visit a professional dental hygienist every three months (Philstrom *et al.*, 2005).

RINSES TO CONTROL PLAQUE AND GINGIVITIS
For a number of people, toothbrushing does not sufficiently control plaque and gingivitis to avoid the onset of periodontal disease. Mouthwashes have been formulated specifically to

support dental hygiene. The most effective rinses recommended for people who have acute gum problems contain chlorhexidine. The teeth may develop a brownish stain and use for longer than 3–4 weeks is not advised. A dentist will be able to remove the stain with professional cleaning.

There has been some concern expressed about the high level of alcohol in some mouth rinses (as high as 25% in some cases), and this has the effect of drying the mouth, which can make gum disease more serious.

CLINICAL CARE OF THE MOUTH

It is a misconception that oral care is common sense (Frenkel, 2003), and one of the most important educational interventions for patients and carers is correct toothbrushing technique and effective denture care.

Procedure: Brushing the teeth
Equipment

- Patient's own toothpaste and toothbrush (preferably small-headed and soft-bristled).
- Pen torch.
- Tongue depressor.
- Receptacle to spit into if not at a sink.
- Chair to sit at if hygiene is being carried out at the sink.
- Clothing protector for the patient.
- PPE.
- Tissues/wipes.
- Clinical waste bag.
- Mouthwash or water to rinse the mouth.
- Prescribed preparations.

NB: The process should take at least 2–3 minutes to ensure thorough brushing.

Action	Rationale
Explain each step of any procedure or examination to the patient and gain their consent	Ensures the patient understands the process and encourages their cooperation
Establish the infection control risk (e.g. does the patient have broken skin, cold sores or any oral infection?). (Immunosuppressed patients should not sit at a communal sink.)	Reduces the risk of infection from water supply
Decontaminate hands and put on selected PPE	Prevents cross-infection
Ensure privacy	
Ensure the patient is sitting comfortably and that their clothes are protected	
Remove any dentures or prosthetics (see 'Denture cleaning' procedure)	
Moisten toothbrush and apply a pea-size amount of toothpaste on the brush	Too much toothpaste can cause a burning sensation in the mouth and can over foam
Stand behind the patient – or sit at the same level as the patient	The nurse should be in a position which allows access to the patient's mouth without crowding the patient
Ask the patient to open their mouth (insert a mouth prop if the patient has difficulty in keeping their mouth open) and, using the categories for oral assessment, inspect the patient's mouth.	Checking the mouth before brushing allows the nurse to identify any sore areas, which need a gentle approach to brushing
Starting at the right side of the patient's mouth, begin to clean the outside surfaces of the upper teeth by tilting the toothbrush at a 45° angle to the teeth at the gum line. Bristles should be pointed towards the gum line	Starting at one side ensures the mouth can be worked over systematically. An angled toothbrush allows improved coverage and plaque removal
Sweep or roll the toothbrush away from the gum line, up the surface of the tooth to the top of the tooth	Prevents bacteria being swept towards the gum, which may increase the risk of gum infection
Use short, gentle sweeping motions (backwards and forwards or circular) until all upper teeth have been cleaned on the outside – pay particular attention to crowns, fillings and difficult-to-reach teeth	Ensures all tooth surfaces are cleaned
Repeat for the inner surfaces of the top teeth	

Action	Rationale
Ask the patient if they wish to stop and spit out residue toothpaste into the receptacle or the sink. Wipe the patient's mouth with a tissue	Prevents the patient feeling uncomfortable from being prevented from spitting. Avoids the patient inadvertently swallowing the fluoride in toothpaste
Rinse brush thoroughly and replace toothpaste	
Repeat the processes for the lower teeth – outside and inner surfaces	Ensures that lower teeth receive the same hygiene measures as the upper teeth
Clean across the surface of the chewing part of the teeth using a forwards and backwards motion	Ensures all tooth surfaces are cleaned
Ask the patient to spit out residue toothpaste. Wipe the patient's mouth with a tissue	Prevents facial soreness from damp skin or toothpaste residue
Rinse the toothbrush and gently brush the surface of the patient's tongue, ensuring that they don't gag on the action	Removes bacteria and freshens breath
Offer the patient water or a measured dose of mouthwash to rinse out the mouth. Wipe the patient's mouth with a tissue	Removes toothpaste residue, which can irritate the mouth if left
If the patient is unable to rinse, use a rinsed toothbrush to sweep over the teeth and moistened foam sticks to wipe the gums and tongue	Removes toothpaste residue
Rinse the toothbrush thoroughly and allow to dry naturally	Prevents bacteria growing on the wet surface
Do not store in a sponge bag or plastic bag	Prevents exposure to bacteria from the air of locker surfaces
Administer (registered nurse if appropriate) any prescribed treatments such as artificial saliva according to instructions	Promotes patient comfort
Apply water-based lubricant or moisturising cream to the patient's lips	Promotes comfort and prevents trauma/cracking of the lips. Reduces the introduction of infection through broken skin
Dispose of all used equipment according to infection control policy	Prevents cross-infection
Decontaminate hands	
Ensure the patient is comfortable and has no other requirements	
Document care according to the patient's care plan and identify need/date for evaluation or reassessment	

Patients who have braces will need special instructions from the orthodontist for managing their oral hygiene. People with braces are often advised to brush in a circular motion. Using dental floss remains important. Poor hygiene while wearing braces can result in discoloration of the teeth after their removal.

MOUTH CARE FOR DEPENDENT PATIENTS

If the intubated patient does not receive effective oral hygiene, bacterial plaque will develop on the teeth within 72 hours, followed by emerging gingivitis.

For some intubated patients, a dental syringe can be used to rinse the mouth. The curved nozzle of the syringe allows fluid to reach difficult areas of the mouth. However, suction using a flexible suction catheter will be required to remove the fluid in order to avoid the patient choking (Berry & Davidson, 2006).

Procedure: Mouth care for the terminally ill or critically ill patient
Equipment

- Denture pot.
- Denture cleaner or toothpaste.
- Denture brush or toothbrush (small-headed with soft bristles).
- Tissues/wipes.
- Gauze swabs.
- PPE.
- Prescribed care, e.g. mouthwash.
- Container of sterile water.
- 10 ml syringe or dental syringe.
- Suction equipment.
- Protective cover for the patient.
- Towel.
- Clinical waste bag.

Action	Rationale
Explain each step of any procedure or examination and gain consent if possible	The patient may not be able to consent but may still be able to hear
Decontaminate hands and put on selected PPE	Prevents cross-infection
Ensure the patient is comfortable and that the environment affords privacy	Dignity must be observed
Check the patient's mouth for any signs of disease, trauma or infection	Assesses for the risk of causing more trauma to a mouth which has damage
If intubated	
Ensure that the endotracheal tube (ETT) is positioned correctly and secure before starting oral hygiene	The risk of accidental dislodgment of the ETT during normal change of tapes is significant; the risk of accidental removal is vastly increased if brushing the patient's teeth while the ETT is not secure.
Patient with own teeth	
Using appropriate moving and handling techniques, position the patient safely (i.e. so they will not choke) with optimum access to their mouth. This will normally require the patient to be lying on their side or with their head turned to the side	Lying on the side or with the face to the side encourages excess fluid to drain out of the mouth and reduces the risk of aspiration into the lungs
Place a protective cover over the patient and the bed linen/pillow	Excess fluid will be absorbed and the patient's comfort will be maintained
Retract the patient's lips either with gauze or insert a wedge	Allows optimum access to the patient's mouth
Brush the teeth (see skill above) using a small amount of fluoride toothpaste or chlorhexidine gel	
Rinse with sterile water from a filled 10 ml syringe or dental syringe; allow fluid to drain from the mouth. Remove any remaining water pooling at the side of the mouth immediately using a flexible suction catheter	Hospital tap water has been identified as a serious source of waterborne nosocomial (hospital-acquired) infections. Special syringes with a curved nozzle are useful for applying mouth rinses to intubated patients. The unique attributes of these syringes allow relative ease of access to all areas of the mouth, including the hard-to-reach posterior region

Continued

Action	Rationale
Using a foam stick or a tongue depressor wrapped with gauze swabs, gently clean the soft palate, soft tissue of the cheeks and the tongue. Discard each foam stick or wrapped tongue depressor after each sweep of the mouth and use a fresh one for the next	This process would also minimise growth of papillae of the tongue, which would normally be eradicated during mastication
Dry the patient's face and lubricate the lips with water-soluble lubricant or moisturising cream	Promotes comfort for the patient
Edentulous patients (no teeth)	
Using appropriate moving and handling techniques, position the patient safely with optimum access to their mouth	Prevents injury or choking
Place a protective cover over the patient and the bed linen	
Retract the patient's lips either manually using gauze or insert a wedge	
Brush the soft palate and soft tissue with either a toothbrush and fluoride toothpaste or foam stick soaked in chlorhexidine gel	Removes debris and prevents injury to the mouth
Rinse with sterile water from a filled 10 ml syringe or dental syringe; allow fluid to drain from the mouth. Remove any remaining water pooling at the side of the mouth immediately using a flexible suction catheter	Prevents choking from the fluid and removes traces of toothpaste which may irritate mucosal lining
Dry the patient's face and lubricate the lips with water-soluble lubricant or moisturising cream	Prevents skin trauma
If the patient has dentures but is unable to wear them, clean the dentures according to the patient's usual routine (see below) and change the water solution/ cleaning solution the teeth are soaking in daily	

Action	Rationale
Reposition the patient if required and ensure that the patient is comfortable with no more care requirements	
Clean away and dispose of used equipment as per local policy. Clean suction machine as per policy	
Evaluate and document care noting any further reassessment needed	

Source: British Society for Disability and Oral Health/Royal College of Surgeons for England (2001)

CARE OF PROSTHETICS: DENTURES AND BRIDGES

It is a myth that visits to the dentist are not required once the teeth have been removed and dentures fitted. The bone that held the teeth in place changes shape once they have been extracted. Therefore, when dentures are originally fitted, they will need to be reassessed in case the bone changes shape to the extent where dentures can no longer be anchored in the mouth. For some people denture fixative is effective, but it is not recommended for long-term use. Fixatives have ingredients that can cause constipation (tragacanth) and erode the enamel of any remaining teeth (kanaya gum).

Dentures are particular breeding grounds for *Candida spp*, in particular bridges and plates. The difficulty with cleaning partial dentures such as these affects the adjacent teeth, which are put at even further risk of decay and plaque build-up. Dentures should be cleaned at least once a day (Preston *et al.*, 2006) with a non-abrasive paste and a soft toothbrush. A soft nail brush with a curved conventional handle can be used by people whose manual dexterity is compromised. General oral hygiene measures are still required as many times daily as for people with their own teeth. People who have dysphagia (swallowing problems) may not manage to remove all food from their mouth while eating (e.g. some people who have had a stroke will 'pouch' food in the side of the face affected by a paralysis). This patient population should be assisted to clean their teeth or dentures and oral cavities after every meal. Not doing so risks food being trapped under the dentures causing abrasions to the gum. Patients who have problems swallowing may also have problems taking conventional oral medication in the form of tablets. Liquid medication should be offered as an alternative but scrupulous oral hygiene is required to prevent burning and/or excoriation of the gums from medication(s).

Soaking the dentures once or twice a week in a **dilute** 2% sodium hypochlorite solution will help to deep clean and remove plaque, but they must not be soaked in hot water. Disinfectants containing bleach should not be used on dentures with any metal components.

COMMON ORAL CONDITIONS IN DENTURE-WEARING PATIENTS
Denture-related stomatitis

Stomatitis is a painful inflammation of the mucous membrane of the mouth (the consequences of untreated stomatitis include sepsis (infection) and ultimately organ failure (Berry & Davidson, 2006). Ulcers or infection noted in the mouth can be directly related to wearing dentures (White, 2000). Other cases include the side effects of medications, the presence of diseases, which oppress the immune system, and anaemia. The frailer and more physically dependent a person is, the more the likelihood that they will have denture-related stomatitis; up to 70% of older people in long-term care homes have been found to have the problem (Frenkel, 2003).

Careful cleaning of the dentures is the most effective prevention. Under the direction of a dental professional, dentures may need to be sterilised in solutions such as dilute hydrogen peroxide. Care must be taken, however, with bridges that have a metal component (Chalmers & Pearson, 2005).

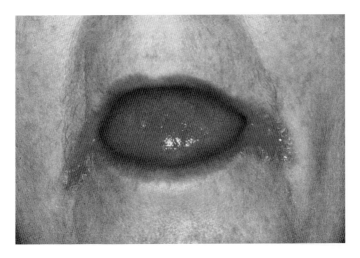

Figure 2.4 Angular cheilitis. Copyright Professor MAO Lewis, Cardiff University. Reproduced with permission.

Angular cheilitis

Yeast infection may be carried via the saliva to the corners of the mouth, which presents as raw skin with cracks and fissures (White, 2000) (Figure 2.4). This can be made worse by the careless insertion of dentures, which can cause the skin to break and bleed. Treatment is with an antifungal topical preparation – usually ointment and an antibiotic cream (Jones, 1998) to prevent *Candida* co-infection.

Procedure: Denture cleaning

Equipment

- Denture pot.
- Denture cleaner.
- Toothbrush/denture brush.
- Tissues/wipes.
- Swabs.
- Protective clothing.

- Prescribed care, e.g. mouthwash.
- Tumbler of drinking water.
- PPE.

Action	Rationale
Explain each step of any procedure or examination to the patient and gain their consent	Ensures the patient understands the process and encourages their cooperation
Decontaminate hands and put on selected PPE	Prevents cross-infection
Ensure the patient is comfortable and the environment affords privacy	Many people dislike being seen without dentures in situ
Ask the patient to remove their top set of dentures and place them into a denture pot	Tissues disintegrate in the moisture of the mouth and may stick to the dentures or teeth
OR	
Using part of a disposable wipe or a gauze swab (not a tissue) loosen the top denture at one side of the patient's mouth and gently pull it forward, place into denture pot	
Ask the patient to remove their bottom set of dentures and place them into a denture pot	
OR	
Using part of a disposable wipe or a gauze swab (not a tissue) using a side-to-side motion, loosen the bottom denture at one side of the patient's mouth and gently pull it forward; place into denture pot	
Offer the patient a tissue with which to wipe their mouth	Removes any saliva which travelled with the teeth
Take the pot with dentures to a sink which is either lined with paper towels or half-filled with water	If the dentures are dropped, they will be less likely to break
Remove dentures from the pot	
Holding dentures over the sink, rinse dentures in tepid water to remove debris	Hot water may damage the material of the dentures and the material of the tooth brush
Using a denture brush or toothbrush, scrub both top and bottom dentures with toothpaste or denture paste or liquid soap and water according to the patient's usual routine	Individualises patient care

Action	Rationale
Rinse dentures thoroughly; check for cracks or sharp edges and that all debris is removed	Removes residue of cleaning agent and prevents irritation of the oral mucosa
Return dentures to the pot – keep the pot dry if returning the dentures to the patient's mouth	
Fill pot with water until teeth are fully submerged if teeth are to be kept out of the patient's mouth, e.g. over night	Dentures will dry out and crack if not stored in moisture
Give a cup of water or mouthwash to the patient. Encourage the patient to rinse their mouth vigorously then void contents into a receiver	Avoids debris from getting trapped under dentures
Offer a paper tissue to the patient to dry their mouth and face	
If the patient is unable to rinse and void, use a rinsed soft toothbrush to clean the tongue and moistened foam sticks to wipe the gums and oral mucosa	Avoids debris from getting trapped under dentures
Before returning the dentures into the patient's mouth, check their mouth for signs of abnormalities, such as redness, painful areas, swelling etc.	Debris may have camouflaged abnormalities
Ask the patient if they have any complaints of abnormalities of their mouth	Patients may have painful mouth, the cause of which may not be apparent
Before returning dentures to the patient ask if denture fixative is needed; follow the manufacturer's instructions for application	The ageing process or disease process may make it more difficult for some patients to retain dentures independently
Return the patient's dentures upper set first. Always insert the teeth at a slight angle (i.e. one side slightly first) and then straighten up when fitting over the gum. Repeat with the bottom set	Avoids overstretching the mouth and causing cracks to the corners of the mouth
Ensure the patient is comfortable and that their teeth are firmly secured	Patients will not be able to eat or speak well if dentures are ill-fitting. Ill-fitting dentures cause abrasions to the oral mucosa
Offer the patient another opportunity to rinse their mouth and/or a drink of water	

Continued

Action	Rationale
Apply lubricant to the lips	Adds to the comfort of the patient
Clear away equipment; rinse the denture brush, allow to dry naturally	
Remove and dispose of PPE and decontaminate hands	
Record any interventions or changes in condition in the patient's care plan and refer to another healthcare professional if required	

GENERAL DENTURE CARE

Patients should be persuaded to remove their dentures into cleaning solution for at least six hours of every 24.

Bacteria in the form of plaque trapped under the dentures causes pain, discomfort and swelling or inflammation under the denture as well as being the cause of candidiasis (thrush), particularly between the denture and the hard palate (roof) of the mouth (White, 2000).

CARING FOR PATIENTS WITH COGNITIVE DEFICITS

People with a profound learning disability, organic brain disease (e.g. dementia), functional disease (e.g. schizophrenia or severe depression) or neurological damage (e.g. head injury) may have difficulty understanding the need for oral hygiene and yet may have the most need of intervention (Nunn *et al.*, 2004).

Particular risks include the effect of prolonged liquid medication use, such as antipsychotics or sedatives, and poor nutrition. Self-neglect of oral health causes problems such as dental caries or gum disease. These conditions if untreated can cause pain, which underpins the reluctance of some people with cognitive difficulties to have any hygiene measures carried out.

Consent is obviously a vital aspect of carrying out any nursing intervention, and any treatment relating to oral hygiene and oral care must be carried out in the patient's best interests. Assessment is vital for these patients to prevent challenging behaviour when carrying out having oral hygiene.

The carers and family are integral to the assessment process as they can provide important information on what processes work best with the patient to achieve teeth cleaning and mouth care.

Certain principles should be observed when using oral health nursing interventions:

- A family member or carer may be more familiar both to the patient and with the normal routine, plus any factors that may hinder care. Therefore, if possible and with the carer/relative's consent, they may carry out oral hygiene for the patient rather than the nursing staff carrying it out.
- The normal procedure must be ascertained, e.g. the patient may not tolerate certain interventions but can be persuaded to use a toothbrush with flavoured toothpaste.
- Any physical intervention to restrain the patient for the procedure should be discussed with the next of kin and the multidisciplinary team and be clearly agreed as being in the patient's best interest.
- Any restraint should be kept to a minimum and must be documented and reviewed at set intervals.
- Any physical intervention should be ceased immediately if the patient shows signs of:
  - Breathing difficulties
  - Physical injury
  - Seizures/convulsions
  - Vomiting
  - Extreme distress
  - Any symptoms of poor circulation (British Society for Disability and Oral Health/Royal College of Surgeons for England, 2001).
- The risk to nursing staff should be assessed and specialist referral made for assistance with management strategies if appropriate.

CONCLUSION

This chapter has highlighted the importance of good oral health for patients and the effects of poor oral hygiene. Good oral health in patients is seen as a marker of good-quality nursing care. Patients require a full oral assessment and individualised nursing care in order to prevent painful conditions. The absence of teeth does not mean that oral hygiene is no longer required and patients can be prone to painful gum conditions and oral infections even when wearing dentures.

REFERENCES

Albino, JE (2000) Factors influencing adolescent cooperation in orthodontic treatment. *Seminars in Orthodontics* **6**(4): 214–223.

Albino JEN (2002) A psychologist's guide to oral diseases and disorders and their treatment. *Professional Psychology: Research and Practice* **33**(2): 176–182.

Berry AM, Davidson PM (2006) Beyond comfort: oral hygiene as a critical nursing activity in the intensive care unit. *Intensive and Critical Care Nursing* **22**(6): 318–328.

Bowsher S, Boyle S, Griffiths J (1999) A clinical effectiveness systematic review of oral care. *Nursing Standard* **13**(37): 31–32.

British Dental Health Foundation (2005) Frequently asked questions. Available at http://www.dentalhealth.org.uk [accessed 1 February 2009].

British National Formulary (2009) *British National Formulary*, 58th edn. Pharmaceuticals Press, London.

British Society for Disability and Oral Health/Royal College of Surgeons for England (2001) *Clinical Guidelines and Integrated Care Pathways for the Oral Health Care of People with Learning Disabilities*. BSDH/RCS, London.

Chalmers J, Pearson A (2005) Oral hygiene care for residents with dementia: A literature review. *Journal of Advanced Nursing* **52**(4): 410–419.

Chamley CA, Carson P, Randall D *et al.* (2005) *Developmental Anatomy and Physiology of Children*. Elsevier, London.

Clarke G (1993) Mouth care in the hospitalized patient. *British Journal of Nursing* **2**(4): 221–7.

Coventry J, Griffiths G, Scully C *et al.* (2000) ABC of oral health: Periodontal disease. *British Medical Journal* **321**(7252): 36–39.

Croucher R (2003) Research Summary: Access to NHS dental care? *British Dental Journal* **195**: 450.

Denton E (1999) Palliative care: Mouthcare: An indicator of the level of nursing care a patient receives? *Journal of Community – Online* **13**(11), http://www.jcn.co.uk/journal.asp?MonthNum=11&YearNum=1999 &Type=backissue&ArticleID=192-36k [accessed 1 March 2009].

Department of Health (2001) *The Essence of Care: Patient-focused benchmarking for health care practitioners*. DH, London.

Department of Health (2005) *Choosing better oral health: An oral health plan for England*. DH, London.

Department of Health (2009) *Further Government Response to the Health Select Committee Report on Dental Services*. The Stationery Office, London.

Dougherty L, Lister SE (eds) (2008) *Royal Marsden Hospital Manual of Clinical Nursing Procedures*, 7th edn. Blackwell Publishing, Oxford.

Feber T (1995) Mouth care for patients receiving oral irradiation. *Professional Nurse* **10**(10): 666–670.

Fiske J, Griffiths J, Jamieson R *et al.* (2000) *Guidelines for Oral Healthcare for Long Stay Patients and Residents*. British Society for Disability and Oral Health, London.

Fitzpatrick J (2000) Oral health care needs of dependent older people: Responsibilities of nurses and care staff. *Journal of Advanced Nursing* **32**(6): 1325–1332.

Fourrier F, Cau-Pottier E, Boutigny H *et al.* (2000) Effects of dental plaque antiseptic decontamination on bacterial colonization and nosocomal infections on critically ill patients. *Intensive Care Medicine* **26**(9): 1239–1247.

Frenkel H (2003) Oral health care: Can training improve its quality? *Nursing & Residential Care* **5**(6): 268–271.

Gallagher JE (1998) Oral health needs: How may they be met? *British Journal of Community Nursing* **3**(1), 25–35.

Griffiths J, Jones V, Leeman I *et al.* (2000a) *Guidelines for the Development of Local Standards for Oral Health Care for Dependent, Dysphagic, Critically and Terminally Ill Patients*. British Society for Disability and Oral Health/ Royal College of Surgeons for England, London.

Griffiths J, Jones V, Leeman I *et al.* (2000b) *Oral Health Care for People with Mental Health Problems: Guidelines and Recommendations*. British Society for Disability and Oral Health/ Royal College of Surgeons for England, London.

Hahn MJ and Jones A (2000) *Mouth Care in Head and Neck Nursing*. Churchill Livingstone, London.

Harker R, Morris J (2005) *Children's Dental Health in the United Kingdom 2003*. Office for National Statistics, London.

Jones CV (1998) The importance of oral hygiene in nutritional support. *British Journal of Nursing* **7**(2): 74–83.

Joshipura K (2002) the relationship between oral conditions and ischaemic stroke and peripheral vascular disease. *Journal of the American Dental Association* **133**(supplement): S23–S30.

Merck (2005) Gingivitis. *Merck Manual*, http://www.merck.com/mmpe/sec08/ch095/ch095c.html, [accessed 1 October 2009].

Miller M, Kearney N (2001) Oral care for patients with cancer: A review of the literature. *Cancer Nursing* **24**(4): 241–254.

Milligan S, McGill M, Sweeney MP *et al.* (2001) Oral care for people with advanced cancer: An evidence-based protocol. *International Journal of Palliative Nursing* **9**(7): 418–426.

NHS Quality in Scotland (2005) *Working with Dependent Older People to Achieve Good Oral Health*. NHS QIS, Edinburgh.

Nunn J, Greening S, Wilson K *et al.* (2004) *Principles on intervention for people unable to comply with routine dental care*. British Society for Disability and Oral Health, London.

Oliver CH, Nunn JH (1996) The accessibility of dental treatment to adults with physical disabilities in the north-east of England. *Special Care in Dentistry* **16**(5): 204–209.

Ottley C (2002) Improving children's dental health. *Journal of Family Health* **12**(5): 122–125.

Pearson LS (1996) A comparison of the ability of foam swabs and toothbrushes to remove dental plaque: Implications for nursing practice. *Journal of Advanced Nursing* **23**(1): 62–69.

Peltola P, Vehkalahti MM, Simoila R (2005) Oral health-related well-being of the long-term hospitalised elderly. *Gerodontology* **22**(1): 17–23.

Philstrom BL, Michalowicz BS, Johnson NW (2005) Periodontal diseases. *Lancet* **366**(9499): 1809–1820.

Preston AJ, Kearns A, Barber MW, Gosney MA (2006) The knowledge of healthcare professionals regarding elderly persons' oral care. *British Dental Journal* **210**(5): 293–295.

Ransier A, Epstein JB, Lunn R *et al.* (1995) A combined analysis of a toothbrush, foam brush and a chlorhexidine-soaked foam brush in maintaining oral hygiene. *Cancer Nursing* **18**(5): 393–396.

Rawlins C (2001) Effective mouth care for seriously ill patients. *Professional Nurse* **16**(4): 1025–1028.

Roberts J (2000) Developing an oral assessment and intervention tool for older people. *British Journal of Nursing* **9**(17): 1124–1127.

Robinson PG, Deacon SA, Deery C *et al.* (2005) Manual versus powered toothbrushing for oral health. Cochrane Database Systematic Review Issue 2. Art. No.: CD002281. DOI: 10.1002/14651858.CD002281.pub2.

Ross A, Crumpler J (2007) The impact of an evidence based practice education programme on the role of oral care in the prevention of ventilator associated pneumonia. *Intensive and Critical Care Nursing* **23**(3): 132–136.

Scottish Executive Health Department (2005) *An Action Plan for Improving Oral Health and Modernising NHS Dental Services in Scotland.* NHS Scotland, Edinburgh.

Scully C, Bedi R (2000) Ethnicity and oral cancer. *The Lancet Oncology* **1**(1): 37–42.

Sharma NC, Galustians HJ, Qaqish J *et al.* (2003) Antiplaque and antigingivitis effectiveness of a hexetidine mouthwash. *Journal of Clinical Periodontology* **30**(7): 590–594.

Sharma NC, Goyal CR, Qaqish JG (2005) Single-use plaque removal efficacy of three power toothbrushes. *Journal of Dentistry* **33**(suppl. 1): S11–S15.

Simons D, Brailsford S, Kidd EAM *et al.* (2001) Relationship between oral hygiene practices and oral status in dentate elderly people living in residential homes. *Community Dentistry and Oral Epidemiology* **29**(6): 464–470.

Singapore Ministry of Health (2004) MoH Nursing clinical practice guidelines: Nursing management of oral hygiene. Ministry of Health, Singapore.

Smith M (2009) Divided by a common tongue: Access. *British Dental Journal* **206**(4): 185.

Southern H (2007) Oral care in cancer nursing: Nurses' knowledge and education. *Journal of Advanced Nursing* **57**(6): 631–638.

White R (2000) Nurse assessment of oral health: A review of practice and education. *British Journal of Nursing* **9**(5): 260–266.

Zulkowski K (2003) How dental status affects healing in older adults. *Nursing* **33**(10): 22.

Care of the Eyes

3

THE IMPORTANCE OF EYE CARE IN GENERAL PATIENT CARE

The eye is the organ of sight which informs us about the surrounding world more than any of the other four senses. We use our eyes in almost every activity we perform, whether for work or leisure. Every day another 100 people start to lose their sight (Royal National Institute for the Blind, 2007). About two million people in the UK report having a sight problem, ranging from being unable to see a friend across the street or read newsprint to being registered as blind. The number of people with sight problems is rising not only because of the rising number of older people but also because the incidence of sight-affecting diseases such as diabetes is also increasing.

Nurses in hospital and primary care settings are expected to become more involved in both the assessment and treatment of people presenting with sight problems, including cataract, glaucoma and low vision (loss of sight) (Ricketts, 2004).

The aim of this chapter is to help the reader understand how to carry out eye care as well as the underpinning rationale(s) for this care.

LEARNING OUTCOMES

After reading this chapter, the reader will be able to:

❑ Describe the anatomy of the eye and the physiology of sight.
❑ Identify common diseases of the eyes during assessment.
❑ Assess for the factors which may impact on sight.
❑ Understand the evidence base underpinning clinical procedures.

❏ Prepare the patient and equipment for eye care procedure(s).
❏ Understand and carry out clinical care of aids relating to the eyes.
❏ Understand and carry out clinical care of the patient's eyes.

Good-quality eye care may not improve the length of a person's life but it has a huge impact on their quality of life (Brown, 2004). The eye allows us to see and interpret shapes, colours and the dimensions of objects by processing the light they reflect or emit.

ANATOMY OF THE EYE

The **eyeball** (Figure 3.1) is protected by a cone-shaped cavity in the skull called the **orbit** (socket); the **eyelids** protect the eye externally by lubricating the eye and spreading tear fluid. They respond reflexively as a defence against possible injury to the eye (Kanski, 2003).

The eye as an organ comprises three connective tissue coatings: the **sclera**, **choroid** and **retina**.

Sclera (white of the eye)

The sclera is the outermost protective film for the eye (Moorfields Eye Hospital NHS Foundation, 2007). At the front of the sclera is the **cornea**, which is transparent and admits light. The cornea curves outwards to allow light entering the eye to bend (refract) focusing onto the retina. The cornea contains no blood vessels but its rich supply of nerves from the optic nerve means that it is extremely sensitive to pain (Moorfields Eye Hospital NHS Foundation, 2007).

Choroid

The choroid forms the middle layer and supplies blood to the rest of the eye. It also absorbs internally reflected light to keep images clear (Watkinson & Seewoodhary, 2007). The front of the choroid has three separate structures: the **iris**, the **ciliary body** (muscles) and the **suspensory ligament**.

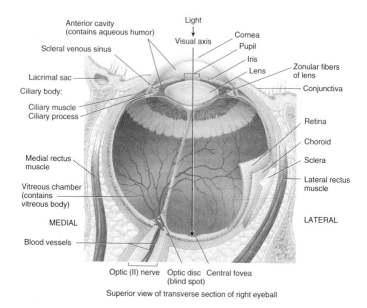

Superior view of transverse section of right eyeball

Figure 3.1 Anatomy of the eye. From Tortora GJ, Grabowski SR (2004) *Introduction to the Human Body: Essentials of Anatomy & Physiology*, 6th edn. Reproduced with permission from Wiley-Blackwell.

The iris is made up of pigmented cells that give the eye its colour. It contains smooth-muscle fibres, which are structured in circular and radial directions. These muscles respond to light in order to control the size of the **pupil**: a circular opening at the centre of the iris (Moorfields Eye Hospital NHS Foundation, 2007). Strong light causes the circular muscle to contract (make smaller) the pupil and so admit less light. The opposite reaction occurs in dim light, but in this instance the radial muscles contract, which pulls the pupil wider to admit more light. The pupil appears black because all the light striking the retina is absorbed and none is reflected out of the eye (Watkinson & Seewoodhary, 2007).

The suspensory ligament, which is attached to the ciliary body, holds the transparent **lens** in place. The lens functions as the second element in the light-focusing system and is situated behind the pupil. The lens changes shape in order to clearly focus on objects which are seen from different distances. For near objects, the ciliary muscles contract, which relaxes the suspensory ligament, and the lens is loosened and bulges (Moorfields Eye Hospital NHS Foundation, 2007). For faraway objects, the suspensory ligament tightens pulling the lens thinner.

The ciliary body, suspensory ligament and the lens also divide the eye into two cavities. The **anterior cavity** (behind the cornea and in front of the lens) is filled with **aqueous humour**, a clear, watery substance, which often leaks out when the eye is injured. **Schlemm's canal**, situated in the sclera, transports the aqueous humour from the anterior chamber into the circulation (Gabelt & Kaufman, 2005). The aqueous humour circulates constantly through the anterior chamber, nourishing the cornea and lens; it flows out through the **trabecular mesh-work**, which is minute spongy tissue situated in the angle where the iris and cornea meet (Glaucoma Foundation, 2007). The fluids in both compartments control the pressure and the shape of the eye. The **posterior cavity** (between the iris, lens and ciliary body) is filled with **vitreous humour**, which is a gelatine-like substance that makes up about 80% of the eye's volume (Moorfields Eye Hospital NHS Foundation, 2007). Vitreous humour maintains sufficient pressure in the eye to prevent the eyeball from collapsing.

The innermost coating is the **retina**, which contains **rod** and **cone cells**. These light-sensitive receptor cells convert the light energy admitted via the pupil into nerve impulses (Moorfields Eye Hospital NHS Foundation, 2007). At the back of the eye is the **macula**, a yellow spot which surrounds the **fovea** (a small indentation at the centre of the macula). This is the area with the greatest concentration of cone cells, and when the eye is directed at an object the part of the image that is focused on the fovea is the image most accurately registered by the brain.

Rod cells contain protein partially derived from vitamin A. Rods are exceedingly responsive to light and enable vision in dim light but cannot distinguish colour. Fine detail and colour come from the cone cells. The cones are responsible for seeing fine detail and colours but are less effective for night vision. Humans have three types of cones, each sensitive to a different colour of light: red, blue and green.

The **optic nerve** (cranial nerve II) pierces the back of the sclera. Within the layers of the retina, light impulses are changed into electrical signals and then sent through the optic nerve, along the **visual pathway**, to the **occipital cortex** at the posterior (back) of the brain. Here, the electrical signals are interpreted (or 'seen') by the brain as a visual image. The **optic disk** is the part of the optic nerve situated on the retina and can be seen on eye examination. This area is also known as the blind spot as it contains no photo-receptors and is therefore insensitive to light (Riordan-Eva & Whitcher, 2007).

The **conjunctiva** is the mucous membrane lining the sclera and eyelids to keep the area moist. Six extra-ocular (outside the eye) muscles control the movement of each eye. Tears are formed by the **lacrimal gland**, found at the front and upper edge of the eye. Tears flow over the eye through the action of blinking to keep it moist and lubricated. Tears also contain a bactericidal enzyme called lysozyme, which cleans the surface of the eyeball and prevents the spread of infection (Thibodeau & Patton, 2008).

VISUAL ACUITY

Binocular vision refers to the ability of both eyes to function by fusing the slightly different images received from the two eyes. This creates good depth perception and allows fine visual judgements to be made when, for example, filling a vessel with liquids. Monocular vision on the other hand means a person has vision in one eye only.

The sudden onset of loss of vision in an eye can result in the patient initially having problems learning to adjust both visually

> **Box 3.1 Enhancing communication ability for a person who has sight impairment in one eye**
>
> - Invite the patient to sit with the majority of the room on their unaffected side.
> - The patient's bed should be placed where the patient has the best view of their surroundings.
> - Approach and talk to the patient from their unaffected side.
> - If walking, the patient should have an unobstructed view of their unaffected side; therefore, the nurse should support the patient from the affected side.
> - The patient may have to move their head awkwardly to compensate for vision loss and to be able to see the face of the person speaking. This can cause people to feel embarrassed.
> - When mobilising, the nurse should provide a commentary on obstacles and unfamiliar sounds.
>
> (*Source:* Houde, 2007; Rushing, 2007)

and psychologically; nurses can use specific strategies to enhance communication and comfort in clinical care (Box 3.1).

THE INFLUENCE OF AGE ON EYE HEALTH AND HYGIENE (LIFESPAN)

Infancy (0–23 months)

The average newborn baby's eyeball is about 18 mm in diameter, from front to back. The eye continues to grow gradually into adulthood where the average eyeball measures around two-thirds the size of a ping-pong ball. At birth, an infant's vision is unfocused except for objects or faces within a very close range – about 30 cm – in front of them. As sight develops, babies will look for longer at patterned objects than single colours, e.g. mobiles above their cots. By two months of age, a baby will focus longer at a smiling face.

Amblyopia is a condition where the development of vision in one eye during childhood is arrested and the brain then fails to understand the images projected by the affected eye. Untreated, this can result in a permanent loss of vision in one eye (Chamley *et al.*, 2005). There are frequently difficulties with close working and it can affect a child's fine-motor ability and educational development.

Childhood (2–12 years)

Myopia (short-sightedness) more often develops in childhood or adolescence when light from an object at distance is focused in front of the retina (i.e. before it gets to the back of the eye) (College of Optometrists, 2009). This causes distance vision to become blurred. Near vision, however, is usually clear. Glasses may need to be worn all the time or just for activities involving distance vision, such as sports.

A squint (strabismus) is also most common in childhood, usually starting between 18 months and four years. In most cases, one eye appears to look straight ahead while the other eye turns inwards (convergent), outwards (divergent) or, less commonly, upwards or downwards (vertical) (Royal National Institute for the Blind, 2008). There is a potential for double vision, as the light is not refracting equally; however, one eye tends to suppress the function of the other. This in turn arrests the development of the eye with the squint, leading to what is commonly referred to as a lazy eye (amblyopia). Occasionally, surgery is required to correct a squint that has not responded to conservative treatment (Royal National Institute for the Blind, 2008).

Adolescence (13–19 years)

Eyesight is one of the senses required to enhance learning. Visual impairments that go unreported by adolescents can affect a teenager's academic ability and impair their social interaction (Lopez, 2002). Females have a significantly higher risk of becoming sight-impaired (World Health Organization, 2004). Some teenagers may show reluctance to wear glasses during their teenage years due to fear of appearing different from their peers. However, glasses are becoming more popular as a fashion accessory and this may have a positive impact on those required to wear them for therapeutic purposes. Contact lenses have become more sophisticated and their use may correct some of the vision impairments in teenagers.

Adulthood (20–64 years)

After age 40, and increasingly after 45, there is a decline in the ability to maintain a clear focus at a near distance (presbyopia). The normal ageing process causes a hardening of the lens and a weakening of the ciliary muscles, which control focusing. This is the reason why many people after the age of 40 years will begin to need glasses for reading and close work (Royal College of Optometrists, 2009).

Older age (65+ years)

In the Western world, age-related macular degeneration (AMD) is the leading cause of impaired sight due to the growing number of people aged over 70 years (World Health Organization, 2004). Another condition associated with ageing – cataracts – remains the leading cause of blindness globally with untreated glaucoma ranking the second-most-common cause of blindness.

THE DEPENDENCE–INDEPENDENCE CONTINUUM INFLUENCING EYE HEALTH AND HYGIENE

The loss of vision to almost any degree in an adult used to being full-sighted compromises function more globally than any other single physical impairment (Mogk *et al.*, 2004). Assisting a patient with visual problems towards independent living in the clinical area includes the following considerations:

- *Mobility:* If the patient has a reduced visual field and poor depth perception, the risk of falls increases in unfamiliar surroundings. This is particularly true for people with cognitive problems (Vu *et al.*, 2005). For those people with bilateral (both eyes) vision loss, falls may result in more severe consequences such as death or having hip replacement surgery. People with reduced vision in both eyes are also more likely to be admitted to long-term care after falls (Wang *et al.*, 2003).

- *Washing and dressing:* Some aspects of meeting fundamental care needs may be difficult for patients and help should be offered sensitively (Chia *et al.*, 2004; Vu *et al.*, 2005). Some clothing colours are difficult to distinguish, e.g. dark blues, blacks and browns (Swann, 2008a).
- *Maintaining a safe environment:* A reduced field of vision may result in the patient bumping into objects or other people. This is particularly true in unfamiliar surroundings and may increase anxiety and reduce confidence (Chia *et al.*, 2004). The patient may be at risk from spilling hot fluids or food.
- *Work and play:* Patients with visual problems can become tired easily when trying to regain independence. Patients may feel isolated within the clinical area (Vu *et al.*, 2005).
- *Communication:*
  - The ability to communicate verbally is impaired in people with low vision. Speech is more difficult to follow if the mouth cannot be seen (Swann, 2008a). Non-verbal cues, which comprise approx 60–90 % of language, are not picked up on.
  - Written communication should be in large enough print to suit the individual, in Braille format or provided through an audio format (Swann, 2008b).
- *Sleeping:* for older people in particular there may be a difficulty entering an area of bright light from a dimmer area, or vice versa. The ageing eye takes longer to adjust to variations in light and the patient may fall or stumble (Swann, 2008a).
- *Nutrition:* Low vision, blindness or vision affected by stroke can cause problems for people trying to maintain their optimum nutritional levels. Difficulty locating food/drinks or cutlery/cups can result in weight loss or dehydration. Accidental spills can cause the patient to feel embarrassed in company and they may refuse food and drinks. Serving foods with contrasting colours (to each other, crockery and tableware) can help (Swann, 2008b).
- *Mental health:* Older people with impaired vision experience various psychological problems, including depression,

confusion, loss of self-esteem and social isolation (Sloan *et al.*, 2005).

PHYSICAL INFLUENCES ON EYE HEALTH AND HYGIENE

Visual difficulties are one of the first signs of multiple sclerosis. Three particular problems can occur. The optic nerve can become inflamed (optic neuritis), causing blurred vision, pain and colour dimming (National Multiple Sclerosis Society, 2002), diplopia (double vision), which can appear without warning, and nystagmus, which is preceded by dizziness. The symptoms are not permanent but may be associated with flare-ups of the condition. Nurses should be aware that demyelinated nerves (i.e. the optic nerve) are very sensitive to heat (National Multiple Sclerosis Society, 2002) and bathing, showering, exercise or a condition which causes the patient to be pyrexial can make the symptoms of optic neuritis worse. The symptoms reduce when the patient is cooled, either with fans, ice packs or cool sponging.

People with diabetes run the risk of developing diabetic retinopathy. This condition, which is symptomless initially, is caused when the blood vessels in the retina become blocked or leaky, or grow randomly and bleed. The retina is damaged and unable to function if untreated. People with diabetes should be encouraged to have eye tests at least twice annually (Diabetes UK, 2008). Treatment is usually by laser, although some people may need surgery.

Patients who have had a stroke are at particular risk of developing a variety of visual problems, many of which do not resolve fully. The common effects include the patient having vision loss of their affected side (homonymous hemianopia) or visual inattention at their affected side, which results in the neglect of any visual stimuli. For example, a person may only eat the food on one half of their plate as they are completely unaware that there is another side to the plate. Damage to the cranial nerve may cause double vision. Nurses must remember that many patients may also have had visual impairment before the onset of a stroke, which can be corrected, and patients should be referred to specialist services (Zihl, 2000).

PSYCHOLOGICAL INFLUENCES ON EYE HEALTH AND HYGIENE

Diseases of the eye can be difficult to camouflage (Dougherty & Lister, 2008), and patients may use tinted glasses, eye protectors or occasionally eye patches to disguise perceived abnormalities. Patients may find that they struggle to cope with the physical impact of their condition and feel disfigured. Isolation can result from the disease process or difficulties in communication (Van Dijk, 2007). Decreased visual function, irrespective of the cause, is associated with a poorer quality of life (Wang *et al.*, 2003; Mogk *et al.*, 2004; Tsai *et al.*, 2004; Knudtson *et al.*, 2005). Low vision has been independently linked to a higher risk of suicide, and general assessment is vital (Box 3.2).

Providing accurate information for patients with visual problems and directing them to specialist practitioners who can provide services and aids for vision is part of the role of the nurse. Even small changes can greatly improve patients' physical and psychological well-being (Tsai *et al.*, 2004). Patients with low vision report that having their condition explained to them and to their families as well as being provided with access to visual

---

Box 3.2 General assessment of patients with low vision

- The patient's own perception of any visual problem.
- The impact of the problem on physical self-care in activities of living, e.g. mobility, maintenance of hygiene, ability to cook, maintenance of personal safety.
- The psychological impact of the problem, e.g. low mood, anxiety.
- The social impact of the problem, e.g. does the patient feel isolated, lonely, do they deliberately avoid social situations?
- The patient's overall perception of any impact of the problem on their quality of life.

(*Source:* Royal National Institute for the Blind, 2007)

---

aids, for example prescription glasses or magnifying implements, has a positive effect on their independence (De Long, 2006). The ability to read and recognise faces were identified as the greatest psychological benefits, as well as having access to aids such as talking watches and books.

SOCIOCULTURAL INFLUENCES ON EYE HEALTH AND HYGIENE

People from some ethnic minorities in the UK may have a particular predisposition to visual problems. Asian children have higher rates of myopia than other racial/ethnic groups, whereas Asian and Afro-Caribbean adults are more likely to develop glaucoma. Sickle cell disease, most common in people of Afro-Caribbean origin, can cause retinal disease (Minassian & Reidy, 2009). Nurses should remember that patients who do not have English as their first language may have even more problems using hospital services and following treatment interventions if they also have low vision.

ENVIRONMENTAL INFLUENCES ON EYE HEALTH AND HYGIENE

Poor air quality causes a rise in pollen levels, which can increase the number of people suffering allergen-related conditions which irritate eyes. The medications prescribed to counteract the condition (e.g. antihistamines) can cause eyes to become uncomfortably dry (British National Formulary, 2009).

People working in dusty conditions may suffer from irritated eyes with excess tear production, itch and burning. Harsh chemicals also irritate eyes but have the added risk of conjunctiva and corneal injury. Workers in inadequately ventilated buildings may find that they develop allergies and dry eyes. Poor lighting and fluorescent lighting – including hospital lighting – can be responsible for eye fatigue, red and sore eyes and blurred or double vision. Glare from sunlight or computer screens can produce similar symptoms and can cause headaches (Healthy Sight Institute, 2008).

POLITICO-ECONOMIC INFLUENCES ON EYE HEALTH AND HYGIENE

Visually disabled people in the UK have on average less income, have less educational and employment opportunities and a more limited social life than sighted people do (International Council of Ophthalmology, 2009). For all people with visual difficulties, certain considerations to aid function and communication are required by nursing staff:

- Written material including patient information leaflets and care plans should be in a format that can be easily read and understood.
- Sight aids, e.g. glasses, contact lenses or magnifying glasses/ sheets, should be maintained in functioning condition and patients encouraged to use them.
- Assessment of the patient's functional ability is important in order to encourage and maintain independence of self-care in the clinical setting.

Referral to specialist optometrist services may also be required for corrective aids [e.g. spectacles (glasses) or contact lenses].

EYE DISEASES/CONDITIONS
Conjunctivitis

Normal defence mechanisms may be broken when infectious agents are introduced to the conjunctiva. Conjunctivitis affects males and females of all ages and cultures. Between 1 and 4% of consultations with primary care health professionals are related to sudden onset of so-called red eye (Sheikh & Hurwitz, 2001).

Signs and symptoms of conjunctivitis vary according to the cause but commonly include:

- Redness.
- Discharge: the patient may have difficulty opening their eyes after sleep due to accumulated matter.
- Irritation.
- Possibly photophobia (light sensitivity).
- Possible swelling of the eyelid.

- Possible blurred vision due to the presence of discharge/excessive tear production.

The causes of conjunctivitis are many and include:

- Viral conjunctivitis.
- Bacterial conjunctivitis.
- Allergic conjunctivitis – characterised by an itch.
- Toxic conjunctivitis.
- Giant papillary conjunctivitis – predominant in contact lens users.

Bacterial conjunctivitis is a microbial infection involving the mucous membrane of the surface of the eye. The normal eye is colonised by flora (bacteria), but alterations in the type of bacteria affecting the eye can lead to the clinical infection of the conjunctiva. Causes include:

- External contamination, e.g. from contaminated hands.
- Spread from adjacent sites, e.g. the other eye.
- Via a blood-borne pathway.

(Sowka *et al.*, 2001)

Assessment of people with conjunctivitis should be carried out sensitively, as there may be a link to sexually transmitted diseases.

Acute bacterial or viral conjunctivitis is usually diagnosed after swabbing for culture and sensitivity. Conjunctivitis is a self-limiting condition in most instances (i.e. the condition will gradually resolve without medical or pharmacological intervention), but patients will need advice as to how to protect themselves and those around them from spreading the condition. However, research suggests that for bacterial conjunctivitis treatment with antibiotic therapy will improve the condition in less time and with few side effects (Sheikh & Hurwitz, 2001). Topical antibiotics may also be prescribed to treat viral conditions as a precautionary measure (British National Formulary, 2009). Eyes should be cleaned (swabbed) before administering any type of prescribed topical treatment.

Procedure: Eye swabbing
Equipment

- Sterile dressing pack.
- Sterile 0.9% sodium chloride for irrigation or sterile water for irrigation.
- Jug of warm water.
- Bath thermometer.
- Receptacle for soiled equipment.

NB: Use an aseptic technique for this procedure.

Action	Rationale
Explain each step of any procedure or examination to the patient and gain their consent	Ensures the patient understands the process and encourages their cooperation
Place water/saline container in a jug of warm water no more than 37°C (measure water temperature with bath thermometer)	Warm water is more comfortable for the patient and provokes less reaction to water near the eye. Warm water removes debris/discharge more effectively
Assist the patient into a comfortable position, ideally a lying position. Head tilted backwards while supported is acceptable	Increased comfort decreases movement
Check the expiry date of the water or saline container	Ensures the preparation is safe to administer
Position the patient with a good light source at the back of them	A light source in front of the patient can cause discomfort
Decontaminate hands	Minimises the risk of cross-infection
Tip sterile dressing pack from its packaging onto the sterile surface and decontaminate hands again	
Open dressing pack and, without touching the sterile pot, pour in the sterile liquid	
Always treat the unaffected eye/less affected eye first	Reduces the risk of transporting infection from one eye to the other
Always bathe lid with the eye closed before commencing swabbing lids	To reduce the risk of damaging the cornea

Continued

Action	Rationale
Ask the patient to look up and, using a slightly moistened low-lint swab, gently swab the lower lid from the nasal corner outwards	Prevents water running down the patient's face and causing discomfort/head movement. Reduces the risk of discharge spreading further into the eye. Reduces the risk of eye-to-eye infection
Avoid touching above the lower lid margin	Avoids discomfort and head movement if the cornea is contacted
Dispose of swabs after each sweep	Avoids reintroducing infection
Repeat the procedure until all debris/ discharge is removed	
Dry lower lid with a new low-lint swab	
Slightly evert (tilt outwards) the upper lid and ask the patient to look down	
Repeat procedure as for lower lid until debris/discharge is removed	
Dry upper lid with a new low-lint swab	
Ensure the patient is returned to a comfortable position with access to the nurse call system	
Remove and dispose of equipment according to local policy	
Decontaminate hands	
Record the nursing intervention and evaluation in the appropriate patient's document	Ensures continuity of care

- Patients with cognitive problems may require help with keeping their head still or may require extra support.
- Patients who are unconscious or ventilated may need additional interventions (Dawson, 2005). During the swabbing procedure, eye drops or ointment may be instilled to keep the eyes lubricated. Polyethylene pads may be applied to the eye for protection and lubrication. Polyethylene covers when compared to lubrication have been shown to reduce the incidence of eye-surface disease (Koroloff *et al.*, 2004). After the procedure, patients may have their eyes taped shut to prevent drying

of the eye or trauma such as corneal abrasions. Taping the eye can occasionally cause unintentional trauma to the eyelid or surrounding skin and can be distressing for relatives to witness.

Corneal abrasion

This is a traumatic injury to the superficial tissue of the cornea (Pavan-Langston, 2002), when a partial or complete removal of the corneal surface produces severe pain, lacrimation (excessive tear production) and blepharospasm (involuntary contraction of the eyelid/excessive blinking). There is a sensation of having a foreign body in the eye made worse by: blinking and involuntary eye movements (Pavan-Langston, 2002). The causes of abrasion are many (Box 3.3) and permanent damage may result (Joyce & Evans, 2006).

Signs and symptoms of corneal abrasion

- Severe pain when moving the eye.
- Lacrimation.

Box 3.3 Common causes of corneal abrasions

Loss of the protective mechanisms, e.g. loss of the blinking ability due to:

- The patient is unconscious/ventilated.
- The patient has been sedated.
- The patient has a neurological disease, e.g. Parkinson's disease, stroke, multiple sclerosis.
- The patient has a learning disability.

  Accidental trauma is commonly caused by:

- Poor contact lens insertion.
- Poor observation of health and safety procedures, e.g. when operating machinery.
- Chemicals splashing into the eye.
- Accidental scratching by fingernails, e.g. rubbing the eye.
- Accidental injury while outside, e.g. tree branches.
- Drying of the eye due to infection.
- The patient resists during any procedure carried out near the eyes.

(Source: Zihl, 2000; Joyce & Evans, 2006)

- Blepharospasm.
- Photophobia (distressed reaction to light).
- Possible blurring of vision.
- Redness of the eye.

(Sowka *et al.*, 2001)

Patients in different care settings can be vulnerable to corneal injury. Those patients in acute care and intensive care units are identified as being at risk because of the effects both of their disease process/trauma and the interventions used within the units (Joyce & Evans, 2006). Any patient who is likely to require assistance with washing may be at risk if nursing staff are not careful when carrying out hygiene care.

Simple corneal abrasions do not usually require padding of the eye, as the healing process is fast. The patient is advised to rest at home and the abrasion usually heals within 24 hours (Sowka *et al.*, 2001).

Dry eyes

Superficial corneal abrasions are also a common result of eye dryness (Joyce & Evans, 2006). Corneal exposure without the protection of tears and blinking can lead to ulceration, perforation and scarring, which may cause permanent damage.

Drying of the eye can be caused by many different factors (Schaumberg *et al.*, 2001; Sowka *et al.*, 2001; Barney, 2002; Joyce & Evans, 2006):

- Inability to close the eye properly.
- The side effects of medications, oxygen therapy and oral contraceptives.
- The ageing process.
- Connective tissue disease, e.g. rheumatoid arthritis.
- Some hormone replacement therapies, including oestrogen therapy.

Despite little evidence beyond expert opinion regarding frequency of nursing interventions or the most effective solutions, the eyes should be kept lubricated (Suresh *et al.*, 2000). A variety of approaches have been used to maintain the tear film and prevent corneal drying and possible injury in general and for people who are unconscious, including:

- Creation of moisture chambers (created by using polyethylene film to cover the eye covers).
- Instillation/application of methylcellulose drops/ointment.
- Use of general lubricants, e.g. liquid paraffin.
- Application of a polyacrylamide gel, e.g. Geliperm.
- Application of a paraffin gauze dressing.
- Instillation of hypromellose drops (artificial tears) (Dawson, 2005).
- Taping the eyelid shut (Watkinson & Seewoodhary, 2007).
- Room humidifiers to add moisture to the atmosphere (Titcomb, 2000).

FOREIGN BODY IN THE EYE

Signs and symptoms of corneal foreign body are similar to those of abrasion but additionally present with:

- Complaints of scratchiness.
- A definite sensation of having a foreign body present.
- The involved eye has a swollen eyelid.
- The conjunctiva and eyeball may also appear irritated.

An eye examination should be carried out to determine whether the foreign body is evident at the surface of or embedded within the cornea – this will usually be carried out by a medical practitioner or a specialist nurse. However, nursing staff may be required to provide aftercare.

Advise rest and information for the patient relating to prevention of future eye injuries. Basic hygiene measures should be communicated and demonstrated to any patient carrying out self-care on discharge (e.g. instillation of eye drops).

CATARACTS

A cataract is a clouding of the lens often as a natural consequence of getting older. Over half of people aged over 65 years will have some cataract development, with most cases treated successfully with surgery. Cataracts develop slowly and are painless. In younger people they can result from an injury, taking certain medication, for example corticosteroids (National Eye Institute, 2006a), long-standing inflammation or illnesses such as diabetes (Royal College of Ophthalmologists and RNIB, 1995).

Aside from older people, those particularly predisposed to cataract formation include people with poorly controlled type 1 diabetes. If normal blood glucose levels are achieved and maintained, cataracts can improve (National Eye Institute, 2006a).

Common symptoms may include the following complaints:

- Because light cannot pass through the clouded lens to the back of the eye, vision is blurred or glasses/contacts lenses seem to be dirty or scratched.
- The cloudiness in the lens may occur in more than one place, causing a double image.
- Bright light or very sunny days may make it more difficult to see.
- As the cataract develops, its centre becomes more and more yellow, resulting in a yellowish tinge to vision.
- Initial awareness of becoming short-sighted.

Once the lens has started to become opaque, the disease progresses with visual ability continuing to deteriorate. This affects the patient's normal living: practical tasks, such as preparing food, or travelling can become impossible; leisure activities can also suffer. Removal is carried out by specialist medical staff.

GLAUCOMA

Glaucoma is a group of eye diseases which are caused in most cases by a back-up of fluid in the eye that increases intraocular pressure. If unrelieved, this pressure causes damage to the ocular nerve and ultimately loss of sight in the affected eye (Glaucoma Foundation, 2007).

Risk factors for glaucoma

- People aged 40 and over – the risk increases with age.
- Those with a family history of glaucoma.
- Those with a visual acuity problem but particularly short-sighted people.
- People with diabetes.

Tests for glaucoma are carried out by optometrists or trained healthcare professionals. Glaucoma sufferers and certain close relatives are entitled to a free eye examination provided by the NHS. Those diagnosed as being at risk of developing glaucoma are also eligible.

Types of glaucoma
Open- (wide-) angle glaucoma
When the trabecular meshwork becomes blocked, pressure builds up, damaging the eye at its weakest point, which is the site in the sclera at which the optic nerve leaves the eye. The optic nerve becomes damaged and the death of the retinal cells and degeneration of the nerve fibres results in permanent vision loss (National Eye Institute, 2006b).

There are rarely clear symptoms relating to glaucoma. The condition is painless and there are no visible changes to the eye. The initial sign that glaucoma may be present is the development of blind spots, particularly in peripheral vision. Only later when the disease has become chronic will central vision be affected. The vision loss is irreversible and therefore permanent (Glaucoma Research Foundation, 2007).

Normal-tension glaucoma
Normal-tension glaucoma is thought to be partly caused by reduced blood flow to the optic nerve, which leads to death of the cells that carry impulses from the retina to the brain. The onset follows the same pattern as for open-angle glaucoma but pressure in the eye is normal. Therefore, keeping intraocular pressure lower than normal is often necessary to prevent further visual loss.

Angle-closure glaucoma

Acute-closure glaucoma is often genetic. It is most common in people who are far-sighted. It is also more prevalent in people of Asian descent.

The anterior chamber is smaller than in the average person and the angle where the cornea and iris meet tends to be less than the usual 45 degrees. The lens increases in size due to normal ageing decreasing the ability of aqueous humour to pass between the iris and lens on its way to the anterior chamber. Pressure builds up behind the iris, further narrowing the angle, which in turn forces the iris against the trabecular meshwork, blocking drainage.

Acute glaucoma

This sudden rise in pressure can occur within a matter of hours and become very painful. Unlike the more chronic conditions, this type of glaucoma presents with signs and symptoms (Sowka *et al.*, 2001; National Eye Institute, 2006b):

- Intense pain possibly causing nausea and vomiting.
- Blurred vision.
- A halo effect around lights.
- Redness of the eye.
- Swelling and dullness of the cornea.
- Sudden onset of sight loss if untreated.

Causes and triggers of an acute glaucoma attack include:

- Being in a dark environment.
- Some eye medications that cause dilating of the pupil, e.g. antidepressants, antihistamines, cold remedies and anti-nausea medication.
- Stress or anxiety.

At the onset of an attack, a person should be encouraged to keep their eye closed to contract the pupil and widen the angle.

Medication in eye drop form can constrict the pupil. If eye drops are combined with medication – and this combination will almost certainly reduce the amount of aqueous fluid produced

– the pressure within the eye can be reduced to safe levels (Glaucoma Research Foundation, 2007).

Surgery will be required in the form of a laser iridectomy to make a small opening in the iris. The entire procedure should take less than 30 minutes and can be done on an outpatient basis. Laser surgery may be performed prophylactically on the other eye, as there is a tendency for both eyes to become affected. Ongoing treatment (e.g. pilocarpine eye drops) can prevent acute glaucoma but does not prevent the chronic attacks (Glaucoma Foundation, 2007).

Many of the conditions above require the use of topical eye preparations to alleviate the consequences of the condition before treatment or to prevent deterioration/recurrence of the condition after treatment.

Procedure: Instillation of eye drops
Equipment

- Prescription sheet.
- Sterile dressing pack and sterile surface.
- Sterile water OR sodium chloride 0.9% for irrigation.
- The prescribed eye drops.
- Swab – low lint (if not supplied in the dressing pack).
- Disposable gloves.
- Waste bag/receptacle for used materials.

Before beginning the procedure, check the prescription sheet and ensure that (Nursing & Midwifery Council, 2008):

- The eye drops are prescribed.
- The correct route for administration and instruction, e.g. 'one eye' or 'both eyes', is written on the drug prescription chart.
- The date for commencement of the prescription is stated.
- The correct strength of preparation to be administered is stated.
- The number of drops of preparation to be administered is stated.
- The date and time(s) for medication administration is clearly written.

- The prescription signature is legible.
- The preparation is within the use by date.

Action	Rationale
Explain each step of any procedure or examination to the patient and gain their consent	Ensures the patient understands the process and encourages their cooperation
Prepare a sterile surface and gather equipment, including PPE	Reduces the risk of introducing dirt into the eye during the procedure
Explain to the patient the possible side effects of the eye drops, e.g. blurred vision, and gain consent to proceed	Ensures that the patient is prepared for unpleasant side effects
Check the name of the patient and their unique hospital number on their identity bracelet against the prescription chart	Reduces the risk of drug error
Ensure from the patient and/or documentation (if patient is unable to answer) that the patient has no allergies to the preparation	Reduces the risk of adverse drug reaction
Check the expiry date of the preparation and the date of opening	Ensures medication is safe to administer
Position the patient with a good light source at the back of them	A light source in front of the patient can cause discomfort
Ask the patient to tilt their head back and look at the ceiling[a]	Ensures eye drops are instilled as intended and minimises loss of preparation out of the eye
Decontaminate hands	Minimises the risk of cross-infection
Tip sterile dressing pack from its packaging onto the sterile surface and decontaminate hands again	
Open dressing pack and, without touching the sterile pot, pour in the sterile water for irrigation	
Remove the top of the bottle of eye drops	
Check the patient's eye for signs of soreness and/or discharge and swab before instilling eye drops (see 'Eye swabbing' procedure)	Increases patient comfort and ensures a clean receptacle for the eye drops
Dampen a sterile swab slightly, using sterile water, and place onto the patient's lower lid	If the swab is too wet, the patient will feel discomfort from drips

Continued

Action	Rationale
Pull down slightly on the swab until the inner of the lower eyelid is exposed	
Ask the patient to look up	
Ensuring that the container of eye drops does not touch the skin, gently drop the prescribed number of drops onto the lower lid	Avoiding skin contact reduces the incidence of infection. Instilling drops directly onto the eye ball causes the patient to overreact
Ask the patient to close their eye and keep the swab in place to absorb any leaking drops	
If the patient complains of a feeling that the drops are running down their throat or the back of the nose, press one finger on the nose just under the eye at the nasal corner	
Remove the swab and check that the patient is feeling no unexpected ill effects	
Repeat the procedure for the other eye if prescribed (check whether separate preparations are prescribed/provided)	Prevents cross-contamination between both eyes
Return the patient to a position of comfort and check that they continue to have no ill effects from the drops. Ensure that the nurse call system is within the patient's reach	
Remind the patient of potential effects from the eye drops	Reduces patient anxiety and increases self-reporting of unusual side effects
Dispose of used equipment according to infection control policy	
Decontaminate hands	
Sign prescription sheet	Maintains an accurate record of care and complies with local drug administration policy
Document additional care in the patient's notes	Provides continuity of care
Observe the patient for adverse effects	

[a]Some patients may be unable, owing to existing conditions, to tilt their heads back without causing pain. In this case, patients should lie on their bed with a light source behind and look back as far as possible (Dougherty & Lister, 2008).

NB: If two or more preparations are prescribed, wait at least five minutes between administering each preparation (Houde, 2007).

Reducing the risk of hospital-acquired infection dictates that the date of opening of the eye drop container should be within one week of the date(s) of administration in clinical care settings. Drops used in the community are often used for up to one month after opening.

Procedure: Instillation of eye ointment
Equipment

- Prescription sheet.
- Sterile dressing pack and sterile surface.
- Sterile water OR sodium chloride 0.9% for irrigation.
- The prescribed eye drops.
- Swab – low lint (if not supplied in the dressing pack).
- Disposable gloves.
- Waste bag/receptacle for used materials.

Before beginning the procedure, check the prescription sheet and ensure that (Nursing & Midwifery Council, 2008):

- The eye drops are prescribed.
- The correct route for administration and instruction, e.g. 'one or both eyes', is written on the drug prescription chart.
- The date for commencement of the prescription is stated.
- The correct strength of preparation to be administered is stated.
- The number of drops of preparation to be administered is stated.
- The date and time(s) for medication administration is clearly written.
- The prescription signature is legible.

Action	Rationale
Explain each step of any procedure or examination to the patient and gain their consent	Ensures the patient understands the process and encourages their cooperation
Explain to the patient the possible side effects of the eye ointment, e.g. blurred vision, and gain consent to proceed	Ensures that the patient is prepared for unpleasant side effects
Check the name of the patient and their unique hospital number on their identity bracelet against the prescription chart	Reduces the risk of drug error
Ensure from the patient and/or documentation (if patient is unable to answer) that the patient has no allergies to the preparation	Reduces the risk of adverse drug reaction
Check the expiry date of the preparation and the date of opening	Ensures medication is safe to administer
Position the patient with a good light source at the back of them	A light source in front of the patient can cause discomfort
Ask the patient to tilt their head back and look at the ceiling[a]	Ensures eye ointments are instilled as intended and minimises loss of preparation out of the eye
Decontaminate hands	Minimises the risk of cross-infection
Tip sterile dressing pack from its packaging onto the sterile surface and decontaminate hands again	
Open dressing pack and, without touching the sterile pot, pour in the sterile water for irrigation	
Remove the top of the bottle of eye ointment	
Check the patient's eye for signs of soreness and/or discharge and swab before instilling eye ointment	Increases patient comfort and ensures a clean receptacle for the eye ointment
Dampen swab slightly and place onto the patient's lower lid	If the swab is too wet, the patient will feel discomfort from drips
Pull down slightly on the swab until the inner of the lower eyelid is exposed	

Action	Rationale
Ask the patient to look up	
Gently squeeze the ointment tube and, holding the tube approximately 2.5 cm (1 inch) above the eye, and starting from the nasal corner, apply a line of ointment along the inner edge of the lower eyelid towards the other side of the eye	Prevents introducing debris/dirt/infection into the lacrimal duct
Ask the patient to close their eye and keeping the swab in place; blot any excess ointment	
Remind the patient that there may be blurred vision on opening the eye	
Remove swab and check that the patient is feeling no unexpected ill effects	
Repeat the procedure for the other eye if prescribed	
Return the patient's head to a position of comfort and check that they continue to have no ill effects from the ointment	
Remind the patient of potential effects from the eye ointment	Reduces patient anxiety and increases reporting of unusual side effects
Dispose of used equipment according to infection control policy	
Decontaminate hands	
Sign prescription sheet	Maintains an accurate record of care and complies with local drug administration policy
Document additional care in the patient's notes	Provides continuity of care
Observe the patient for adverse effects	

[a]Some patients may be unable, owing to existing conditions, to tilt their heads back without causing pain. In this case, patients should lie on their bed with a light source behind and look back as far as possible (Dougherty & Lister, 2008).

NB: When using both ointments and drops, use the ointment AFTER the drops (Dupree, 2007).

CARE OF AIDS TO VISION

Many conditions that are not necessarily disease processes can impact on vision (e.g. long-sightedness). The majority can be corrected with the use of glasses or contact lenses. Part of the nurse's role is to help the patient maintain good channels of communication, and this is not possible for a patient who depends on prescribed eye aids, unless they are well maintained.

Contact lenses

Contact lenses have obvious cosmetic advantages and many people have better vision with contact lenses than they do with spectacles. Although there is a slight increase in the risk of eye infection, with proper care the risk is minimised (North Glasgow University NHS Division, 2002).

There are usually two types of contact lenses available:

- Rigid gas-permeable.
- Soft.

Within these categories, there are numerous variations:

- Daily wear.
- Daily disposables.
- Extended wear (overnight use).
- Continuous wear, ranging from one to six nights or up to 30 days.

Of all contact lens types, soft extended-wear contact lenses carry the smallest risk of corneal abrasion but have a far greater risk of infection than the soft daily wear type and gas-permeable lenses (Martin & Barr, 1997).

It is an important part of admission assessment to determine what type of lens is used by the patient and their routine for maintenance and lens care. Although nurses cannot prescribe or fit contact lenses initially for the patient, they are ideally placed to support patients in coping with their use (Stollery *et al.*, 2005) and preventing complications (Box 3.4).

Box 3.4 General care of contact lenses

Follow the care and disinfection regime as advised by the opthamologist, including:

- Discarding unused cleansing solution after 28 days.
- Avoiding the use of tap water for cleansing.
- Not using saliva as a moisturiser or cleanser.
- Keeping equipment scrupulously clean.
- Removing lenses for a spell each day to allow the cornea to breathe.
- Removing lenses at night if not the extended-use variety.
- Keeping hands free from hand cream or scented soap.
- Avoiding water sports while wearing lenses.
- Removing lenses on signs of irritation and/or infection.

(*Source:* Martin & Barr, 1997)

The use of contact lenses needs to be considered carefully with the administration of certain medications. For some people, local anaesthetic drops may be used to reduce the initial pain of inserting lenses (Downie *et al.*, 2003). However, some medications instilled topically into the eye can be absorbed by soft lenses and this can lead to localised toxic reactions (Downie *et al.*, 2003).

Contact lens use may also be contraindicated with medications that work systemically (are metabolised by the body), including:

- Medicines which reduce tear production, e.g. antihistamines, beta blockers and diuretics.
- Medicines which increase tear production, e.g. ephedrine.
- Medicines which reduce blink frequency, e.g. hypnotics and muscle relaxants.
- The oral contraceptive can cause problems for some contact lens wearers.

Procedure: Insertion of contact lenses
Equipment

- Clean surface.
- Contact lenses in their own storage case.

NB: Use a clean technique for this procedure.

Action	Rationale
Explain each step of any procedure or examination to the patient and gain their consent	Ensures the patient understands the process and encourages their cooperation
Decontaminate hands	
Ensure that your fingers are clean and dry	Dry fingers facilitate handling, as soft contact lenses tend to stick to wet fingers
Remove one lens from the storage case (whichever the patient normally inserts first)	
Rinse the lens with the recommended neutralising and/or moisturising solution	Removes all traces of dirt/dust
Place the lens on the tip of your index finger with the curved side next to the skin	
With your other hand, gently pull the patient's upper lid upwards and ask the patient not to blink	Blinking interferes with the insertion of the lens
With the middle finger of your inserting hand, gently pull down the lower lid	
Ask the patient to look up and gently lower the lens on to the lower white of their exposed eye	
Release both eyelids and ask the patient to close their eye for a moment	
Ask the patient to blink several times	Centres the lens over the eye
Ensure that there is no irritant on insertion	Ensures that no debris has been introduced
Repeat the procedure for the other lens	
Ensure the patient is comfortable and has access to the nurse call system	
Wash and dry the lens box	Provides clean storage of the lenses on removal. A dirty case is a major source of infection
Clear away equipment safely	
Decontaminate hands	

(*Source:* Ramponi, 2001; North Glasgow University NHS Division, 2002)

Procedure: Removal of soft contact lenses (Figure 3.2)
Equipment

- Clean surface.
- Cleaning solution for lenses as recommended by ophthalmologist.
- Clean storage box for lenses.

NB: Use a clean technique for this procedure.

Action	Rationale
Explain each step of any procedure or examination to the patient and gain their consent	Ensures the patient understands the process and encourages their cooperation
Decontaminate hands	
Ensure that the lens is centred in the patient's eye	Facilitates easy removal and reduces the risk of trauma
Ask the patient to look up and gently pull down the lower lid with the middle finger	
Using the index finger of the same hand, lower the lens onto the lower white part of the patient's eye	
Gently squeeze the lens between your thumb and index finger	Bends the lens slightly to allow removal without injuring the eye
Remove the lens from the eye, taking care not to scratch the lens	
Follow the lens care procedure recommended by the ophthalmologist	
Place the lens safely in the patient's lens storage box	Prevents damage to the lens from dust/debris
Repeat the procedure for the other lens	
Check the patient's eyes for signs of irritation	
Ensure the patient is comfortable and has access to the nurse call system	
Clear away equipment safely	
Decontaminate hands	

(*Source:* Ramponi, 2001; North Glasgow University NHS Division, 2002)

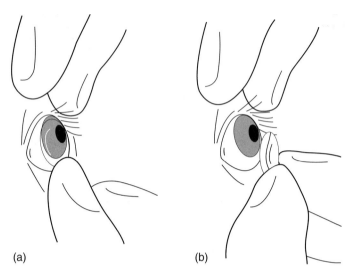

(a)   (b)

Figure 3.2 Removal of soft contact lenses. (a) Moving a soft lens down the interior part of the sclera. (b) Removing a soft lens by pinching it between the pads of the thumb and index finger. From Dougherty L, Lister S (2008) *The Royal Marsden Hospital Manual of Clinical Nursing Procedures*, 7th edn. Reproduced with permission from Wiley-Blackwell.

Procedure: Removal of hard contact lenses
Equipment

- Clean surface.
- Cleaning solution for lenses as recommended by ophthalmologist.
- Clean storage box for lenses.

NB: Use a clean technique for this procedure.

Action	Rationale
Explain each step of any procedure or examination to the patient and gain their consent	Ensures the patient understands the process and encourages their cooperation
Decontaminate hands	
Using one finger placed on the outside corner of the patient's eye, gently draw the skin back towards the ear	The patient's eyelids will lie tightly against the eyeball
Cup your other hand against the patient's cheek below the eye	Prevents the lens from falling onto a surface and becoming scratched
Ask the patient to blink to allow the lens to exit from the eye	
If the lens does not move, gently pinch the patient's upper and lower lids together	Loosens the lens and allows easier removal
On catching the lens, place it safely into the storage container	Prevents damage to the lens from surfaces
Repeat the procedure for the other lens	
Check the patient's eyes for signs of irritation	
Ensure the patient is comfortable and has access to the nurse call system	
Clear away equipment safely	
Decontaminate hands	

The patient should always be encouraged to have a pair of spectacles available for when lenses are not practical to wear. Glasses or spectacles should be maintained in working order to facilitate optimum communication for the patient while in the clinical area (Box 3.5).

PROSTHETIC EYES

Many eye conditions can cause discomfort or pain and possible disfigurement. Eye conditions range from mild symptoms (e.g. slight redness) to tumours of the eye globe and surrounding structures (Van Dijk, 2007; Dougherty & Lister, 2008). Treatment is based on cure and preserving sight, but if the tumour is extensive enucleation (removal of the eye globe) and insertion of a

---

Box 3.5 General care of glasses

- If appropriate, ensure that the patient's glasses are identified through labelling – *if lost, the patient becomes more dependent + replacement glasses are expensive.*
- Patients with cognitive or physical difficulties may need to have different pairs of glasses distinguished for varying needs (e.g. reading glasses should be easily distinguishable from glasses used for distance) – *increases independence and ensures that the patient is safely wearing the correct glasses if mobilising within the clinical area.*
- Glasses should be washed daily in warm soapy water and dried with a soft clean, non-abrasive cloth – *glasses can harbour infection and dirt.*
- Lenses must be polished at least twice a day. To do this, simply breathe on them and rub them with a felt or impregnated cleaning cloth. Appropriate cloths are usually supplied with glasses – *improves vision and avoids scratching the lenses.*
- Cloths should be kept clean and not used for any other purpose – *prevents the spread of infection and keeps the lenses cleaner and scratch free.*
- Encourage patients to keep their glasses in the case when not in use and not to rest them on hard surfaces – *prevents scratching of the lenses and reduces the risk of glasses being mislaid.*
- Check whether the patient's glasses are a good fit, i.e. do they sit straight? If not, refer to a specialist for reassessment – *if glasses are twisted out of shape, vision will not be as clear.*
- Ensure that the patient has a good light source – *this helps the patient's eyes to function better.*

(*Source:* Swan, 2008b)

---

prosthetic (false) eyeball may become necessary (Dougherty & Lister, 2008). Although older people and people with learning disabilities have an increased likelihood of developing eye conditions, younger people, including children, are susceptible to traumatic eye disorders (Marsden, 2002) that can result in accidental eye loss.

Procedure: Removal of a prosthetic eye (Figure 3.3)
Equipment

- Clean flat surface.
- A storage box for the eye.

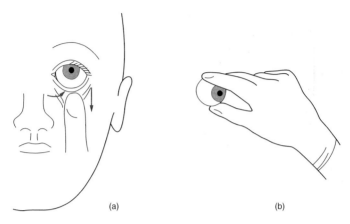

(a)   (b)

Figure 3.3 Removal of a prosthetic eye. From Dougherty L, Lister S (2008) *The Royal Marsden Hospital Manual of Clinical Nursing Procedures*, 7th edn. Reproduced with permission from Wiley-Blackwell.

NB: Use a clean technique for this procedure.

Action	Rationale
Explain each step of any procedure or examination to the patient and gain their consent	Ensures the patient understands the process and encourages their cooperation
Ensure the patient is sitting or lying comfortably	
Decontaminate hands	
Ask the patient to look upwards and gently push the lower lid down with the index finger until the lower ledge of the prosthesis can be seen	Exerting slight pressure below the eyelid overcomes the suction, enabling the prosthesis to be removed
Ask the patient to look downwards and cup your hand under the patient's eye socket	The prosthesis will slide out downwards over your index finger, allowing it to be caught in the other hand
Clean the eye socket with sterile 0.9% sodium chloride and low-linting gauze	Prevents damage to the eye and reduces the risk of introducing dirt with the eye

Continued

Action	Rationale
The prosthesis can now be washed, and either reinserted or placed in its container	
Clear away used equipment according to local policy	
Decontaminate hands	
Evaluate and document care	

(*Source:* Moorfields Eye Hospital NHS Foundation, 2007)

Should the prosthetic eye require storage for any length of time, it should be kept in a solution of 0.9% sodium chloride to prevent it drying out (Downie *et al.*, 2003).

Procedure: Insertion of a prosthetic eye
Equipment

- Clean flat surface.
- Prosthetic eye in a storage box.

NB: Use a clean technique for this procedure.

Action	Rationale
Explain each step of any procedure or examination to the patient and gain their consent	Ensures the patient understands the process and encourages their cooperation
Ensure the patient is sitting or lying comfortably	
Wash the prosthetic eye with running warm water and liquid soap, washing-up liquid or simple shampoo and rinse thoroughly	Prevents any mucous and debris re-entering the eye socket
Place the prosthetic eye in a clean storage box until it's ready for insertion	Prevents damage to the eye and reduces the risk of introducing dirt with the eye
Decontaminate hands	
Holding the prosthesis between the thumb and middle finger of your right hand (if right-handed)	

Action	Rationale
Place the index finger on the centre of the prosthesis and with the middle finger of the left hand gently lift the upper eyelid	
Ask the patient to look down and insert the dotted edge of the prosthesis under the lid. When it is halfway in, let go of the lid, but continue to hold the prosthesis in position with the index finger of your right hand	Prosthetic eyes normally have four coloured dots along the top edge
Ask the patient to look up and gently pull down the lower lid with your other hand until the prosthesis slips under its edge. The prosthesis is now in place	
Ask the patient if the eye feels comfortable. Gently correct the eye's position by stroking and rotating it	
Ensure the patient is returned to a comfortable position with access to the nurse call system	
Remove and dispose of equipment according to local policy	
Decontaminate hands	

CONCLUSION

This chapter has reviewed some care issues for patients who either have low vision as a result of a disease process or have conditions which will require eye hygiene and care of aids for sight. Low vision and conditions which impair eyesight can reduce quality of life. The eye is a fragile organ, and careless nursing can cause more trauma to the eyes. Prescribed care can alleviate eye conditions or prevent deterioration.

REFERENCES

Barney NP (2002) Can hormone replacement therapy cause dry eye? *Archives of Ophthalmology* **120**(5): 641–642.

British National Formulary (2009) *British National Formulary*, 58th edn. Pharmaceuticals Press, London.

Brown M (2004) Patient Expectations Regarding Eye Care Focus Group Results, *Evidence Based Eye Care* **5**(1): 56–57.

Chamley CA, Carson P, Randall D *et al.* (2005) *Developmental Anatomy and Physiology of Children*. Elsevier, London.

Chia E-M, Wang JJ, Rochtchina E *et al.* (2004) Impact of bilateral visual impairment on health-related quality of life: The Blue Mountains Eye Study. *Investigative Ophthalmology and Visual Science* **45**(1): 71–76.

Dawson D (2005) Development of a new eye care guideline for critically ill patients. *Intensive and Critical Care Nursing* **21**(2): 119–122.

De Long SK (2006) Getting help: A low vision patient survey. *Eyecare Business Magazine* **20**(8), http://www.eyecarebiz.com/article.aspx?article=51176, [accessed 12 October 2009].

Diabetes UK (2008) Retinopathy, http://www.diabetes.org.uk/Guide-to-diabetes/Complications/Long_term_complications/Retinopathy/, [accessed 1 March 2009].

Dougherty L, Lister SE (eds) (2008) *Royal Marsden Hospital Manual of Clinical Nursing Procedures*, 7th edn. Blackwell Publishing, Oxford.

Downie G, MacKenzie J, Williams A (2003) *Pharmacology and Medicines Management for Nurses*, 3rd edn. Elsevier Churchill Livingstone, London.

Dupree D (2007) The Macula Centre: Home care instructions for eye drops or ointment, http://www.maculacenter.com/Meds/EyeDrops.htm, [accessed 12 October 2009].

Gabelt BT, Kaufman PL (2005) Changes in aqueous humor dynamics with age and glaucoma. *Progress in Retinal and Eye Research* **24**(5): 612–637.

Glaucoma Foundation (2007) About glaucoma, http://www.glaucomafoundation.org/about_glaucoma.htm, [accessed 5 October 2009].

Glaucoma Research Foundation (2007) Treating glaucoma, http://www.glaucoma.org/treating/index.php, [accessed 5 October 2009].

Healthy Sight Institute (2008) Environmental factors affecting health sight, http://www.healthysightinstitute.org, [accessed 4 October 2009].

Houde S (2007) *Vision Loss in Older Adults*. Springer Publishing, New York.

International Council of Ophthalmology (2009) Vision for the future, part 2: Economic benefits of ophthalmologic care: Socioeconomic Aspects of blindness, available at http://www.icoph.org/prev/costsoc.html [accessed at 3 October 2009].

Joyce N, Evans D (2006) Eye care for patients in the ICU. *American Journal of Nursing* **106**(1): (suppl. 'Critical Care Extra') 72AA–72DD.

Kanski J (2003) *Clinical Ophthalmology*. Blackwell Publishing, Oxford.

Knudtson MD, Klein BEK, Klein R *et al.* (2005) Age-related eye disease, quality of life, and functional activity. *Archives of Ophthalmology* **123**(6): 807–814.

Koroloff N, Boots R, Lipman J *et al.* (2004) A randomised controlled study of the efficacy of hypromellose and Lacri-lube combination versus polythene/cling wrap to prevent corneal breakdown in the semiconscious intensive care patient. *Intensive Care Medicine* **30**: 1122–1226.

Lopez R (2002) *The Teen Health Book: A parents' guide to adolescent health and well-being*. WW Norton, New York.

Marsden J (2002) Ophthalmic trauma in the emergency department. *Accident and Emergency Nursing* **10**(3): 136–142.

Martin S, Barr O (1997) Preventing complications in people who wear contact lenses. *British Journal of Nursing* **6**(11): 614–619.

Minassian D, Reidy A (2009) Future sight loss in the decade 2010 to 2020: An epidemiological and economic model: A report prepared for the RNIB, http://www.rnib.org.uk/aboutus/Research/reports/eye-health/Documents/FSUK_Report_2.doc, [accessed 7 October 2009].

Mogk MD, Lylas G, Mogk M (2004) 'Saving Lives: The Impact of Vision Loss in Later Life'. Presented by Dr Mogk at the Pfizer Ophthalmology Therapeutic Area Conference, 25 March 2004, http://www.mdsupport.org/library/savinglives.html, [accessed 3 March 2009).

Moorfields Eye Hospital NHS Foundation (2007) Anatomy of the eye, http://www.moorfields.nhs.uk/Eyehealth/Anatomyoftheeye, [accessed 15 March 2009].

National Eye Institute (2006a) Resource guide: Cataract, http://www.nei.nih.gov/health/cataract/cataract_facts.asp, [accessed 9 March 2009].

National Eye Institute (2006b) Resource guide: glaucoma: Causes and risk factors: Who is at risk for glaucoma? http://www.nei.nih.gov/health/glaucoma/glaucoma_facts.asp#2e, [accessed 5 October 2009].

National Multiple Sclerosis Society (2002) Vision problems, http://www.nationalmssociety.org/download.aspx?id=65 [accessed 7 March 2009].

North Glasgow University Hospital NHS Division (2002) *Clinical Procedure Manual: Section A: General procedure guidelines, 1.3.* NHS Strathclyde, Glasgow.

Nursing & Midwifery Council (2008) *Standards for Medicines Management*, NMC, London.

Pavan-Langston D (2002) *Manual of Ocular Diagnosis and Therapy (Spiral Manual Series)*, 5th edn. Lippincott Williams & Wilkins, Philadelphia.

Ramponi DR (2001) Eye on contact lens removal: Learn how to master this delicate procedure with skill and confidence. *Nursing* **31**(8): 56–57.

Ricketts B (2004) *First Report of the National Eyecare Services Steering Group*. Department of Health, London.

Riordan-Eva P, Whitcher J (2007) *Vaughan & Asbury's General Ophthalmology*, 17th edn. McGraw-Hill, London.

Royal College of Ophthalmologists and RNIB (1995) Understanding eye conditions related to diabetes, http://www.rcophth.ac.uk/docs/college/patientinfo/UnderstandingEyeConditionsRelatedtoDiabetes.pdf, [accessed 15 November 2008].

Royal College of Optometrists (2009) Eyesight problems, http://www.college-optometrists.org/index.aspx/pcms/site.Public_Related_Links.Eyesight_Problems.Eyesight_Problems_home/, [accessed 5 October 2009).

Royal National Institute for the Blind (2007) Research, http://www.rnib.org.uk/xpedio/groups/public/documents/publicwebsite/public_researchstats.hcsp, [accessed March 2009].

Royal National Institute for the Blind (2008) Childhood squint, http://www.rnib.org.uk/xpedio/groups/public/documents/publicwebsite/public_childhood_squint.hcsp#P2_16, [accessed 5 March 2009].

Rushing J (2007) Helping a patient who's visually impaired. *Nursing* **37**(8): 29.

Schaumberg DA, Buring JE, Sullivan DA *et al.* (2001) Hormone replacement therapy and dry eye syndrome. *Journal of the American Medical Association* **286**(17): 2114–2119.

Sheikh A, Hurwitz B (2001) Topical antibiotics for acute bacterial conjunctivitis: A systematic review. *British Journal of General Practice* **51**(467): 473–477.

Sloan FA, Ostermann J, Brown DS *et al.* (2005) Effects of changes in self-reported vision on cognitive, affective, and functional status and living arrangements among the elderly. *American Journal of Ophthalmology* **140**(4): 618–630.

Sowka AW, Gurwood AS, Kabat AG (2001) Handbook of Ocular Disease Management, http://www.revoptom.com/HANDBOOK/oct02_sec2_4.htm, [accessed 7 October 2009].

Stollery R, Shaw ME, Lee A (2005) *Ophthalmic Nursing*. Blackwell Science, Oxford.

Suresh P, Mercieca F, Morton A, Tullo A (2000) Eye care for the critically ill. *Intensive Care Medicine* **26**(2): 162–166.

Swann J (2008a) Understanding visual and auditory loss. *Nursing & Residential Care* **10**(4): 195–197.

Swann J (2008b) Visual impairments: Assistive devices. *Nursing & Residential Care* **10**(3): 138–139.

Thibodeau GA, Patton KT (2008) *Structure and Function of the Body*, 13th edn. Mosby Elsevier, St Louis.

Titcomb LC (2000) Eye disorders: Over-the-counter ophthalmic preparations. *Pharmaceutical Journal* **264**(7082): 212–218.

Tsai S-Y, Chi L-Y, Cheng C-Y *et al.* (2004) The impact of visual impairment and use of eye services on health-related quality of life among the elderly in Taiwan: The Shihpai Eye Study. *Quality of Life Research* **13**(8): 1415–1424.

Van Dijk K (2007) Providing care for children with low vision. *Community Eye Health Journal* **20**(62): 24–25.

Vu HTV, Keeffe JE, McCarty CA *et al.* (2005) Impact of unilateral and bilateral vision loss on quality of life. *British Journal of Ophthalmology* **89**(3): 360–363.

Wang JJ, Mitchell P, Cumming RG *et al.* (2003) Visual impairment and nursing home placement in older Australians: the Blue Mountains Eye Study. *Ophthalmic Epidemiology* **10**(1): 3–13.

Watkinson S, Seewoodhary R (2007) Common conditions and practical considerations in eye care. *Nursing Standard* **21**(44): 42–47.

World Health Organization (2004) Magnitude and causes of visual impairment, http://www.who.int/mediacentre/factsheets/fs282/en/, [accessed in 8 March 2009].

Zihl J (2000) *Rehabilitation of brain disorders after brain injury*. Psychology Press, Hove, East Sussex.

Ear Care

4

THE IMPORTANCE OF EAR CARE

One in five people has hearing loss that is often of gradual onset (Royal National Institute for Deaf People (RNID), 2004). Hearing loss is not always recognised until it impacts on a person's ability to converse effectively (Tolson *et al.*, 2002). The RNID estimates that two million people in the UK have hearing aids and a further three million people have a degree of hearing loss. Only 75% of people with hearing aids use them regularly (Royal National Institute for Deaf People, 2009a). Nurses are likely to discover people with undiagnosed hearing loss, particularly in very young children or older people. The RNID (2004) suggests that the presence of deafness can be an indicator of other disabilities, particularly in older people.

The aim of this chapter is to help the reader understand how to carry out care of the ears and the underpinning rationale(s) for care.

LEARNING OUTCOMES

After reading this chapter, the reader will be able to:

❑ Describe the anatomy of the ear and the physiology of hearing.
❑ Identify common diseases of the ears during assessment.
❑ Assess for factors impacting on hearing.
❑ Prepare the patient and equipment for the procedure(s).
❑ Understand and carry out clinical care of the patient's ears.
❑ Understand and carry out clinical care of prostheses relating to hearing.
❑ Understand the evidence base underpinning clinical procedures.

The ear is a sensitive and easily damaged organ (NHS Quality Improvement Scotland, 2006) and many aspects of ear care must be undertaken by a registered nurse who has been educated and demonstrated competence in specialised clinical skills.

ANATOMY OF THE EAR

The ears are the organs of hearing and balance constructed in three sections: the **outer ear**, the **middle ear** and the **inner ear** (Figure 4.1).

The outer ear (auricle or pinna)

This organ situated on the side of the head is commonly recognised as the ear and comprises **fibro cartilage** covered by **epithelium** (skin). The skin of the ear is covered by fine hairs which become denser in the **tragus** (covers the ear canal), particularly

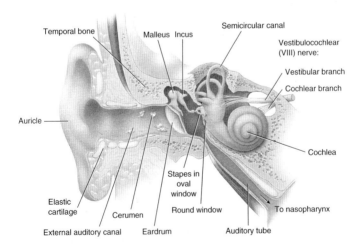

Frontal section through the right side of the skull
showing the three principal regions of the ear

Figure 4.1 Anatomy of the ear. From Tortora GJ, Grabowski SR (2004) *Introduction to the Human Body: Essentials of Anatomy & Physiology*, 6th edn. Reproduced with permission from Wiley-Blackwell.

in males after middle age. The **lobule** (ear lobe) forms the lowest part of the ear and is made up of fibro-fatty tissue (Thibodeau & Patton, 2008).

The ear canal (external auditory meatus)

The ear canal extends from the outer ear to the **tympanic membrane** (eardrum). The canal is lined with a thin layer of epithelium tightly attached to the structures beneath it. Any inflammation tightens the tissue causing pain. The **ceruminous glands** are situated in the cartilaginous part of the meatus and produce cerumen (wax). Sounds enter the outer ear travelling down the ear canal until they reach the tympanic membrane. On reaching the eardrum, the sound vibrates and is passed into the middle ear.

The middle ear

The middle ear is an air-filled cavity (**tympanic cavity**) linking the outer ear and inner ear. The outer and middle ears are separated by the eardrum (**tympanic membrane**). It is also connected to the back of the **throat/nasopharynx** by a small passage called the **Eustachian tube**. The Eustachian tube keeps air pressure on both sides of the eardrum equal. Usually, the walls of the tube are collapsed but actions such as swallowing and chewing open the tube to allow air in or out as needed to maintain equal pressure. The eardrum vibrates when struck by sound waves.

Within the middle ear are three tiny **ossicles** (movable bones). These smallest bones in the body link together, stretching from the eardrum to the **cochlea** (the hearing organ situated within inner ear). Vibrations from the outer ear pass to the **malleus** (hammer), which pushes the **incus** (anvil), which pushes the **stapes** (stirrup). The oval window which leads to the inner ear sits immediately behind the stapes and vibrates when 'struck' by the stapes. These bones conduct sound waves mechanically through the middle ear to the inner ear.

The inner ear

The inner ear is connected to the middle ear by two membrane-covered outlets: the **oval window** and the **round window**.

The inner ear consists of a **bony labyrinth** (maze of fluid-filled tubes), running through the temporal bone of the skull. Within the bony labyrinth is a second series of fluid-filled tubes, called the **membranous labyrinth** in which the actual hearing cells are situated. The inner ear has two functions: hearing and balance, which are controlled by different parts within the inner ear.

The cochlea (hearing)

The cochlea is a spiral-shaped fluid-filled chamber. When sound vibrations enter the cochlea, the fluid moves and hair-like nerve cells trigger an electrical pulse in the **auditory nerve**. Hair cells pick up different frequencies of sound depending on where they are positioned in the cochlea. The round window disperses the pressure generated by the fluid vibrations, pushing or expanding as needed. The vibrations or nerve impulses travel over the **cochlear nerve** to the **auditory cortex** of the brain, where they are interpreted as sound.

The vestibular system (balance)

Three semicircular canals lie perpendicular to each other. Fluid flows within the semicircular canals in response to movement which stimulates hair cells to move. The vestibular system is also filled with fluid and has five small sections. Each of these sections detects head movement in a different direction. The fluid within these sections moves in response to shifting of the head. In a similar way to the hair-like cells in the cochlea, they turn the mechanical movement into an electrical signal before sending the information to the brain along the cranial nerve. This information is used in conjunction with vision and sensors situated within joints (e.g. knees and hips for maintenance of balance). This information stimulates reflex actions to respond to a potential loss of balance. For example, fluid moving in the semicircular canals triggers leg or arm reflex movements to restore balance.

Cerumen (wax)

A normal amount of earwax is healthy, as the skin of the ear canal depends on the earwax for lubrication, protection against bacteria and prevention of insects and dust getting into the ear (Action on ENT Steering Board, 2007). The ear canal skin moves at the rate of 33 mm each year, shedding dead skin cells, which become part of the earwax situated at the entrance of the ear canal (Waugh & Grant, 2004).

Cerumen is a mixture of an oily substance containing **sebum** (fatty acids), sweat and dead skin; it is slightly acidic, which means it has antifungal and bactericidal properties (Rodgers, 2003). It has a wet, sticky form common to Caucasian and Afro-Caribbean people but a dry flaky form in Oriental people, who also tend to dryness of the outer ear. The **ceruminous glands** are found in the cartilaginous part of the ear canal; they increase their secretions in response to the stress hormones adrenalin, noradrenalin released during stress, pain and fear (Burton & Doree, 2003).

Wax is also milked along the ear canal by the action of the lower jaw during chewing and speaking. The colour of cerumen varies from golden yellow to black, and the consistency may be thin and oily or hard. Exposure to water may cause the plug to expand and impact. Excess production may be linked to dietary habits or hereditary factors (Roeser & Ballachanda, 1997).

HEARING LOSS

There are around nine million people in Britain with some degree of hearing loss and an estimated two million who have hearing aids but only about 1.4 million who actually use them (Royal National Institute for Deaf People, 2007). Deafness can be present from birth or acquired but is highly likely to impact on communication ability.

There are four main types of hearing loss:

- Conductive.
- Sensorineural.
- Mixed hearing loss.
- Central hearing loss.

Conductive hearing loss

The conduction of sound transmitted to the middle ear is reduced. This may involve cerumen (wax) build-up or rigidity of the ossicles in the middle ear. Accumulation of cerumen is common in older people as the ceruminous glands decrease in number and the wax secreted becomes drier and more easily impacted. Conductive hearing loss can also be caused by infections or a middle ear tumour.

Sensorineural hearing loss

Hearing loss results from damage to any part of the inner ear or the neural pathways to the brain. Patients with sensorineural hearing loss also find it difficult to filter background noise, for example in ward situations or outpatient clinics (Royal National Institute for Deaf People, 2009c). It can result from genetic causes, from systemic disease, substances introduced into the ear which are toxic or prolonged exposure to loud noise. Side effects of common medications including antibiotics, non-steroidal anti-inflammatory drugs (usually painkillers) and diuretics can cause sensorineural hearing loss, as can chemotherapy and antimalarial drugs.

Mixed hearing loss

This is a combination of conductive and sensorineural impairment common as part of the ageing process and secondary to disease processes.

Central hearing loss

Central hearing loss occurs when auditory processing is disrupted at the brain. While the ear function and hearing process may remain normal, the person with central hearing loss may lose the ability to interpret language.

Accurate diagnosis and treatment for any hearing loss require advanced assessment and intervention strategies and should be handled by an expert in this area (Wallhagen *et al.*, 2006).

THE INFLUENCE OF LIFESPAN ON EAR HEALTH AND HYGIENE

Infancy (0–23 months)

Listening is part of learning for newborn babies. As babies respond to voices and sound while focusing on the facial expressions of the speaker, pathways in the brain are being formed. Newborns can recognise the voices of their main carers and will turn their heads in the direction of sound (Chamley *et al.*, 2005). Babies from 1–3 months will respond to being spoken to by using facial expressions and body movements. Screening babies for deafness will usually occur at around 8 months and testing is carried out round the baby's responses to sound which is produced out of the baby's line of vision. By the age of 1 year the baby will begin to babble and use two-syllable words (e.g. 'da-da').

Nothing should ever be put in a baby or child's ear to clean them. Babies and young children are more susceptible to ear infections if fed lying down rather than sitting, if they use a dummy or if the parent/carer(s) smoke (BUPA, 2008).

Childhood (2–12 years)

Conversation starts around the age of 2 in the form of small sentences. Speech delay, or failing the hearing screening test, may indicate glue ear in children, which will require referral to an ear, nose and throat (otolaryngology) specialist.

As children begin to attend nursery and mix with other children, the incidence of ear infections will increase. Although ear infections may not be infectious, the common cold that causes the ear infection is and normal infection control procedures should be undertaken to prevent cross-infection.

Seventy-five per cent of all middle ear infections will occur in children under the age of 10 years (SIGN, 2003). Many children may have residual fluid in their middle ear after a cold but this will resolve within a few weeks.

Adolescence (13–19 years)

There are no major differences between ear care for older children and teenagers. However, more teenagers may seek multiple piercings of their ears than younger children, with increased infection risks. Infections are usually caused by poor infection control during the process, frequently touching the site with unclean hands or earring posts that are too tight. Earrings that are too tight may reduce the blood supply to the area, which increases the risk of skin trauma and infection. Dangling earrings increase the risk of ear trauma, especially if worn while playing sports.

New research may suggest that teenagers are at risk of losing their hearing through the prolonged use of music players such as MP3 players and iPods (Fligor & Cox, 2004). Advice for teenagers should include: keep the player at a volume (no more than 60% of the maximum) where voices can still be heard when earplugs are worn and ration the amount of time using earplugs while listening to music to no more than one hour per day. The time can be extended if earphones are used rather than earplugs.

Adulthood (20–64 years)

Most people will not notice any alteration to their hearing before the age of 60. However, for some people who are exposed to noise as part of their occupation or hobby, ear protectors should be worn. Signs of having been exposed to noise which could cause damage include ringing in the ears or sounds being heard as flat or dull (National Institute for Occupational Safety and Health, 1996). Generally, increased exposure to noise in a variety of ways has caused a 26% increase in reported hearing loss.

Adults are not at the same risk of acquiring ear infections as children are, but when they do get them the complications include residual fluid in the ear, pressure, pain and temporary hearing loss.

Older age (65+ years)

The normal ageing process can cause changes in the ear that affect hearing acuity. Presbycusis is the most common form of sensori-neural hearing loss associated with ageing. The hair-like cells in the cochlea deteriorate over the years and are unable to vibrate effectively, meaning that quiet sounds are not heard. It is typically gradual, affects both ears and characterised by high-frequency hearing loss (Bagai *et al.*, 2006). Many consonants, such as *t*, *p* and *s*, are high-frequency sounds, while the vowels are low-frequency sounds. Consonants convey most of the information needed to make words distinct and comprehensive. As a result, louder speech will not necessarily help, because the high-frequency consonants remain inaudible. Hence, some older adults with presbycusis say that they can hear but not understand what is being said. Hearing aids are useful in the management of presbycusis.

THE EFFECT OF DEPENDENCE IN ACHIEVING EAR CARE

Patients who have conditions which impair their ability to move freely in bed are susceptible to pressure sores on the ear. Pressure caused by lying in bed is exacerbated by the use of a hearing aid and therefore it becomes difficult to communicate spontaneously with the patient using verbal communication only. A temperature which results in sweating can cause maceration of the skin on the ear if hygiene is not maintained. Even patients who have a history of vomiting or those with conditions where excess saliva is produced or saliva is not swallowed easily can be prone to maceration of the ears from damp pillowcases.

There is a high overall incidence of hearing difficulties in people with learning disabilities. These are due to a variety of factors, including genetic tendencies to deafness (e.g. fragile X syndrome); structural abnormalities within the organ and neural complications can reduce hearing, which may further complicate communication difficulties for this population.

PHYSICAL FACTORS INFLUENCING EAR HEALTH, HEARING AND HYGIENE

Hearing loss has many causes (Box 4.1). The ear as an organ is easily damaged, particularly the eardrum and middle/inner ear. The organ is largely self-cleaning in people with normal ear physiology and hygiene is easily maintained in the absence of physical or mental impairment. However, failure to maintain basic ear hygiene can result in hearing impairment and organ damage. People with dermatological conditions of the periauricular skin (skin on and around the ear) or scalp are also susceptible to dry, painful or broken skin, which can cause pain and increase the risk of infection.

Box 4.1 Causes of hearing loss

Childhood

- Prenatal (before birth): maternal rubella (German measles).
- Perinatal (during birth): premature birth/birth injury.
- Postnatal (after birth): childhood infections, e.g. mumps.

Later childhood/adulthood

- Repeated infections, e.g. otitis media (middle ear infection).
- Disease processes, e.g. Ménière's disease, meningitis.
- Medication side effects, e.g. aspirin.
- Earwax build-up.
- Ongoing exposure to noise, e.g. machinery, loud music through earphones.

PSYCHOLOGICAL FACTORS INFLUENCING EAR HEALTH, HEARING AND HYGIENE

Hearing loss can prevent people from communicating effectively and can result in social withdrawal and isolation. Hearing difficulties can increase depression, cause anxiety and even family conflict (Tolson *et al.*, 2002). Many people fail to seek help for hearing loss because of the gradual nature of its onset, as people may adapt without consciously realising they are losing hearing ability. Additionally, there remains a perception that there is a social stigma attached to wearing a hearing aid and therefore people may be reluctant to seek professional help (Rees, 2004).

SOCIOCULTURAL FACTORS INFLUENCING EAR HEALTH, HEARING AND HYGIENE

Several factors for consideration have been identified for people from ethnic minorities in relation to those who are deaf or have low hearing. There have been comments that sign language and lip-reading services for people do not take into account language barriers; this results in deaf people feeling marginalised among their families and ethnic groups (Ahmad *et al.*, 1998). Patients with pierced ears or multiple piercings require additional cleaning of the holes to avoid infection.

ENVIRONMENTAL FACTORS INFLUENCING EAR HEALTH, HEARING AND HYGIENE

It is important to remember that, as well as listening, most people find it helpful to watch people's faces and lip-read when in conversation. Most people lip-read in certain circumstances, for example in noisy social situations where it is difficult to be heard. Gestures and expressions are an important part of communicating, and patients may rely more on reading a nurse's body language and gestures even when using a hearing aid (NHS Quality Improvement Scotland, 2005).

POLITICO-ECONOMIC FACTORS INFLUENCING EAR HEALTH, HEARING AND HYGIENE

There continues to be debate around deafness as a disability. Some people who have been deaf from birth feel strongly that being deaf is part of their cultural identity rather than a disability. This leads to a dichotomy of being 'deaf' as a biological impairment and 'Deaf' as a separate culture (Corker, 1998). This may not be so true of people who become hard of hearing or deaf in later life, although deaf people have been known to feel part of a Deaf community at any time in their lives.

People belonging to Deaf communities have sign language as their first language. In Britain, British Sign Language (BSL) is the means of communication.

While there is an acknowledgement that services for deaf people are developing and funding is improving (Ahmad *et al.*, 1998), services for those who are hard of hearing remain poorly organised and poorly funded. NHS services have also been found wanting in meeting the needs of people with hearing problems: almost half (42%) of deaf and hard of hearing people find it difficult to communicate with NHS staff. This rises to 77% of people who use sign language. Often there are no BSL interpreters available as translators (Scottish Council on Deafness, 2009).

MAINTAINING NORMAL HYGIENE OF THE EAR

Production of excess earwax is not associated with poor personal hygiene, but ear hygiene needs to be carried out carefully to avoid

---

Box 4.2 Fundamental ear hygiene

- Never insert any implements such as cotton buds into the ear.
- To dry/clean the outside of the ear, use a dry tissue or alcohol-free baby wipes around and behind the ear after the patient has showered/bathed.
- Use a soft disposable damp cloth to gently wipe around the cartilaginous area of the ear.

If there are signs of inflammation or the patient is complaining of any discomfort:

- Keep the ears dry, avoiding any entry of water; shampoos and soaps may be irritating to the skin.
- When washing hair, use cotton wool coated in petroleum jelly or ear plugs placed at the entrance to both ear canals.

---

causing damage to the ear (Box 4.2). However, public awareness of this is low and leads to misguided attempts to remove wax with such instruments as cotton swabs and hairpins. Aside from traumatising the skin, these actions often contribute to increased wax production and impaction and can also impair the self-cleansing mechanism of the organ (Burton & Doree, 2003). Using implements to clean ears can also cause trauma to the lining of the ear canal or the eardrum itself.

COMMON EAR CONDITIONS
Cerumen impaction
Cerumen impaction is the most common of ear, nose and throat (ENT) problems, despite the ear being a self-cleaning organ. Impaction is caused by compressed wax in the ear canal, completely obstructing the lumen (Browning, 2004). Cerumen tends to be drier and harder in older people, plus the ageing process can decrease the mobility of the ear canal. The ear becomes blocked with wax with a degree of hearing loss. (See Box 4.3 for other risk factors.) A small amount of cerumen in the external meatus is normal. The absence of any wax may be a sign that dry skin or infection has interfered with normal wax production (Browning, 2004). Trying to remove earwax using cotton buds,

---

Box 4.3 Risk factors for cerumen impaction

- Narrow or abnormal ear canal.
- Large amount of hairs in the ear canal.
- Presence of benign bony growths in the external auditory canal (osteomata).
- Presence of a dermatological disease around the ear or scalp.
- Production of hard wax, as this is more likely to become impacted.
- Previous history of recurrent impacted wax.
- Learning disability: the reason for this is not known.
- Recurrent otitis externa.
- Use cotton buds for ear cleaning.
- Use of a hearing aid or ear plugs.
  (*Source:* Baer, 2005; Harkin, 2005; Action on ENT Steering Board, 2007**)**

---

matchsticks or other implements can push a plug of cerumen deeper into the canal. This can result in dull hearing and even pain if the wax is pushed against the eardrum. Rubbing the ear canal with implements can stimulate the glands to make more wax and can make the problem worse.

The use of ear drops to soften and disperse the wax is the first line of treatment and is the least likely to cause damage. Clinical evidence suggests that the use of ear drops is recommended over no intervention unless the person has a perforated tympanic membrane. There are several over-the-counter ear drops available to aid the removal of earwax, including those which claim to dissolve wax. Proprietary wax-removing agents have not been shown to be more effective than saline or water (Hand & Harvey, 2004). Many proprietary preparations contain organic solvents that are not recommended, because of the risk of irritation and inflammation of the external ear canal. (Somerville, 2002). Simple remedies include coconut, almond and olive oil. However, owing to the potential of nut allergy, olive oil is usually the preferred choice. Ideally, the olive oil should be inserted into the ear twice per day for one week (Action on ENT Steering Board, 2007). This encourages the natural movement of cerumen out of the ear by lubricating and softening the earwax. The successful use of ear

---

Box 4.4 Suggested circumstances for referral to specialists in patients with cerumen impaction

- Significant itching of the ear.
- Discharge from the ear (otorrhoea).
- Swelling of the external auditory meatus (possible infection).
- Anyone has (or is suspected to have) a chronic perforation of the tympanic membrane.
- Any history of ear surgery.
- There is a foreign body in the ear canal.
- Ear drops have been unsuccessful and irrigation is contraindicated.
- Irrigation is unsuccessful.
- Pain.
- Sudden complete hearing loss.
- Vertigo.

(*Source:* Aung & Mullay, 2002)

---

drops may result in no further intervention(s) – such as aural toilet (ear syringing or irrigation) – being required (Harkin, 2005).

Referral to specialists may be required in certain circumstances (Box 4.4). Although there is little evidence to guide practice regarding when to remove earwax, excessive earwax should be removed in the following circumstances (NHS Quality Improvement Scotland, 2006; Action on ENT Steering Board, 2007; Roland *et al.*, 2008):

- If the tympanic membrane must be viewed for diagnostic reasons and is occluded by wax.
- If an ear mould is required for a hearing aid.
- If earwax causes a hearing aid to whistle.
- If earwax occludes the tympanic membrane and any of the following conditions are also present:
  ○ Tinnitus
  ○ Earache
  ○ Vertigo
  ○ Hearing loss
  ○ A cough connected to presence of earwax.

There is a risk with instillation of any ear drops that the patient may suffer temporary deafness or, if the drops are too cold when they are instilled, dizziness.

Procedure: Instillation of ear drops

Once they have been prescribed by the doctor, ear drops can be given by any nurse who is competent to administer them.

Equipment

- Prescription sheet.
- The prescribed ear drops.
- Cotton wool or gauze swabs.
- Tray/receptacle for disposing of used materials.
- Wear protective clothing – gloves and apron.

Before beginning the procedure, ensure that (Nursing and Midwifery Council, 2008):

- The correct route for administration and instruction, e.g. one or both ears, is written on the drug prescription chart.
- The date for commencement of the prescription is stated.
- The correct strength of preparation to be administered is stated.
- The number of drops of preparation to be administered is stated.
- The date and time(s) for medication administration is clearly written.
- The prescription signature is legible.

Action	Rationale
Explain each step of any procedure or examination to the patient and gain their consent	Ensures the patient understands the process and encourages their cooperation
Decontaminate hands	Minimises the risk of cross-infection
Check the name of the patient and their unique hospital number on their identity bracelet against the prescription chart	Reduces the risk of drug error

Continued

Action	Rationale
Ensure from the patient and/or documentation (if patient is unable to answer) that the patient has no allergies to the preparation	Reduces the risk of adverse drug reaction
Check the expiry date of the preparation	Ensures medication is safe to administer
Drop the bottle of liquid into a small jug of warm water (which has been measured by a water thermometer as being 37°C) for two minutes	
Ask the patient to lie on their opposite side from the ear to be treated **OR** If patient is to remain seated ask them to tilt their head to the side opposite from the ear to be treated – approximately 90° if tolerated	Increases patient comfort and reduces possible reaction of dizziness
Pull the cartilaginous part of the pinna backwards and upwards[a]	Straightens the ear canal and increases access
Squeeze the prescribed number of drops into the external canal	
Ask the patient to remain in their position for 2–5 minutes	Keeps the medication in place to increase the therapeutic action
If there is any oozing from the ear, mop with the cotton wool or gauze	Increases patient comfort
Repeat procedure for the other ear if prescribed	
Dispose of used cotton wool or gauze according to policy	
Return patient to a position of comfort and check that they have no ill effects from the drops and are comfortable	
Decontaminate hands	
Sign prescription sheet	Maintains an accurate record of care and complies with local drug administration policy
Document additional care in the patient's notes and identify any referral required	Provides continuity of care
Observe patient for adverse effects	

[a]Children: pinna should be pulled backwards only (Royal College of Paediatrics and Child Health, 2003)

Children, people with learning disabilities or older people with cognitive impairment may require to be held gently while having ear drops instilled. It may be easier for them to lie on their back in a slightly upright position but with their head tilted to the side. Cotton wool should not be placed at the entrance to the ear canal, as it acts as a wick for the oil and as a barrier to the natural migration of cerumen out of the ear.

If the symptoms of ear impaction persist, ear irrigation may be considered, providing that there are no contraindications for the procedure. (This is an extended role and is outwith the remit of this book.) If irrigation is unsuccessful, ear drops can be used for a further 3–5 days and/or the patient may require ENT referral.

COMMON HEALTH CONDITIONS OF THE EAR
Otitis externa (inflammation of the skin of the ear canal)
The skin of the ear canal becomes inflamed due to one or more of the following causes (NHS Scotland, 2005):

- The lining or the outer ear canal has been irritated by scratching or introduction of a foreign body, e.g. cotton bud.
- Presence of a skin condition such as eczema.
- A fungal/viral/bacterial infection is present.
- Trauma.

Risk factors for developing the condition include (Sander, 2001):

- Being in warmer temperatures/high humidity.
- Swimming.
- Hearing aid use.
- Use of, e.g., protectors at work – raised infection risk.

Treatment interventions include (Block, 2005):

- Remove or treat any precipitating or aggravating factors.
- Prescribe or recommend analgesia for pain relief.
- Prescribe a topical ear preparation for seven days (may include antibiotic and/or corticosteroid preparations).
- Specialist referral may be required for cleaning of the ear canal or insertion of an ear wick.
- Advice may be required for prevention of recurrence.

Box 4.5 Signs and symptoms of otitis media

- Low-grade pyrexia.
- Earache.
- Lethargy.
- Irritability.
- Children and babies may pull at their ears and be distressed.
- Decrease, dullness or loss of hearing.
- Discharge from the ear (symptom that the eardrum has perforated, especially if there is relief of pain).
- Inflammation of the external ear (pinna) may or may not be present.

(*Source:* Mills, 2008; Stevens, 2008)

Otitis media (middle ear infection)

Otitis media is an infection or inflammation of the middle ear usually caused by a viral or bacterial infection. The source of the infection is usually from the mucous membrane of the pharynx in the throat, which spreads through the auditory tube (Bluestone, 2000). Because this tube is so much shorter in children up to the age of about 8 years, they are more susceptible to otitis media than adults are (Chamley *et al.*, 2005). Otitis media can be acute or chronic, but as its symptoms (Box 4.5) may not be severe, it may remain untreated for a long time, possibly causing more damage than an acute infection (Bluestone, 2000).

The infection can prevent the Eustachian tube from opening as it should and air cannot reach the middle ear. When this happens, the middle ear can fill up with fluid that can become thick, like glue. This problem is called glue ear (or otitis media with effusion). The build-up of fluid in the middle ear reduces the movement of the eardrum and ossicles, resulting in a loss of hearing. The changes in pressure caused by the build-up of fluid can be painful. If the build-up of fluid is extreme, the eardrum (tympanic membrane) can rupture.

Most people recover without medical intervention or antibiotics, but taking painkillers such as paracetamol or ibuprofen reduces pain and temperature. Medical intervention and antibiotic therapy may be required for repeated or chronic glue ear in children (Williamson *et al.*, 2006). To allow air into the middle ear and prevent a build-up of fluid, the surgical decision may be made to insert grommets (small tubes for ventilation) into the eardrum. This is a temporary measure and is rarely required past childhood.

Perforated eardrum(s)

Perforated eardrums can be caused by untreated otitis media or by other serious ear infections. Head injuries, loud explosions (loud enough to alter the pressure in the eardrum) or inserting foreign bodies into the ear can also cause a perforation. These normally heal spontaneously and without medical interventions with any hearing loss being temporary (Cook & Walsh, 2005). More serious and long-lasting damage can be treated by surgery. A myringoplasty would be performed where a skin graft is used to seal the perforation.

Tinnitus

'Tinnitus' is the word for the noises heard in ears or the head that do not come from a tangible outside source. It has been described as buzzing, ringing, whistling, humming or hissing. Tinnitus can affect one or both ears, the middle of the head or an area that is difficult to pinpoint. The noises can vary from low through medium to high-pitched and can be intermittent or continuous. About 10% of the adult population experience a continuous mild degree of tinnitus but many find themselves hypersensitive to normal background noise (hyperacusis).

The exact cause of tinnitus is not fully understood, but risk factors include (Daugherty, 2007):

- The ageing process (although children are rarely affected, tinnitus is not exclusive to older people).
- Prolonged exposure to loud noise.
- Psychological conditions (anxiety, emotional upset).
- Head injury.
- Medication side effects, including ototoxic medications (toxic to the ear), e.g. aspirin.

- Middle or inner ear infection.
- High blood pressure (hypertension).

Although some forms of tinnitus are untreatable, the condition may not be permanent. Patients should be encouraged to keep active but nursing staff should be alert for signs of depression (British Tinnitus Association, 2000). Strategies which can reduce the effects include:

- Medication review.
- Exercise, weight loss and a salt-reduced diet to reduce blood pressure/antihypertensive medication if required.
- Tinnitus retraining therapy is often provided by audiologists.
- Increasing personal coping through psychological therapy, e.g. cognitive therapy/stress management/relaxation techniques.
- Use of noise generators, which produce soothing sounds, e.g. water. These come in different forms, e.g. pillow speakers and radios.
- Use of ear protectors to avoid continuous noise damage.
- Avoid prolonged use of MP3 players, iPods, personal stereos or articles requiring use of earplugs/headphones.
- The use of soothing background noise (not via earplugs), e.g. music to counteract the internal noise from tinnitus.

True vertigo

The symptoms of true vertigo may include a very strong feeling that the room is moving or of a sense that one is moving or spinning when stationary. This feeling may worsen on actual movement, accompanied by nausea and vomiting (Yardley, 1994). These episodes of vertigo are not constant but come and go.

- Sense of movement.
- An illusion of spinning and circling.
- Worsened with head movements.
- Nausea/vomiting.
- Episodes come and go.
- Rhythmic eye movement (nystagmus).

Ménière's disease

Ménière's disease is a rare inner ear disorder of the hearing and balancing mechanisms that brings spontaneous episodes of vertigo that can last minutes or hours (Osbourne, 2009). The onset of the condition usually affects only one side, but around 30% of people with Ménière's develop bilateral problems (Warrell *et al.*, 2003). There may be some intermittent hearing loss in the affected ear and the person's balance is often affected. Other accompanying symptoms include:

- An increase in tinnitus.
- A sense of fullness in the affected ear.
- Sudden onset of vertigo, which may increase in severity.
- Nausea/vomiting.

(Ménière's Society, 2009)

The disease is most common between the ages of 20 and 50 and can be distressing, because attacks are unpredictable, recurrent and can last between several hours and a day (Osbourne, 2009). It is a progressive disease, which means that the symptoms may gradually become more intense and of longer duration (Yardley *et al.*, 1998).

ASSESSMENT AND SCREENING FOR HEARING IMPAIRMENT/EAR CONDITIONS

Assessment or screening for hearing impairment isn't routinely performed, even for older people in inpatient settings. However, nursing staff, if alert, can identify people with potential hearing difficulties through observant care and gentle exploration of hearing ability with the patient (Box 4.6).

The screening version of the Hearing Handicap Inventory for the Elderly (HHIE-S) (see Appendix 4.1) assesses the psychosocial impact of hearing loss for people living in the community. It is a short (five-minute) 10-item questionnaire; the higher the HHIE-S score, the greater the potential problems associated with hearing loss. Referral to audiology is recommended for individuals scoring 10 or higher on the inventory (Demers, 2004).

Box 4.6 Observations and questions to detect hearing problems

- Does the patient cup their hand behind or nearly behind their ear?
- Does the patient tilt their head or lean towards the speaker when listening?
- Does the patient often ask people to repeat what has been said?
- Does the patient have the volume very high on the television or radio?
- Does the patient complain of ringing, roaring or buzzing in their ears?
- Does the patient misinterpret words or fail to respond to being spoken to?
- Does the patient fail to join in with others' conversations?
- Does the patient look withdrawn?

Any of these signs should prompt further exploration with the patient. Simple questions are as sensitive in detecting mild to moderate hearing impairment as audiometric testing. Assessment of the patient's perspective of any problems is also important in order to tailor care and plan nursing interventions. Ask the patient:

- Do you have a hearing problem?
- Do you feel you have a hearing loss?
- Is this problem becoming worse?
- Are both ears causing problems?
- Under what circumstances is it most difficult to hear?
- Do you feel you have any other problems with your ears?

(*Source:* Gates *et al.*, 2003; Wallhagen *et al.*, 2006)

Assessment/screening questions

NHS Quality Improvement Scotland (2005) suggests assessment/ screening questions to form a history for the healthcare professional, which comprise:

- Have you had ear surgery?
- Have you experienced ear problems before?
- Have you had perforated eardrum(s) previously?
- Do you suffer from tinnitus?
- Do your ears ever itch?
- Do you use cotton buds in your ears?
- Do you avoid getting water in your ears? If so, how?
- Are you aware of any allergies?
- Have you any skin complaints?
- Do you swim? If so, how often?

If there are clinical indications of inflammation in, or surrounding, the ear, also ask the patient if they have made any changes to toiletries or detergents.

According to the RNID (2004a), more than one in five patients with hearing difficulties have left a consultation with a doctor unsure what is wrong with them. Nurses should be aware that the quality of their communication with a patient who has hearing impairment could affect not only the information and understanding a patient has while in a care situation but also the patient's quality of life (Rees, 2004). Therefore, communicating verbally with a patient should be perceived as a skill.

Procedure: Verbal communication with a patient who has a hearing impairment

Action	Rationale
Approach the patient within their field of vision	The patient is not startled, which will lower anxiety
Ensure that any hearing aid(s) are in place and functioning	Improves the patient's ability to communicate
Ensure that glasses, if needed, are worn	Visual cues can improve understanding of speech
If necessary, invite the patient to a quieter location	Minimises background noise; provides increased privacy
Ensure any light is on your face and not on the patient's	Shadows on the face can reduce visual cues for the patient
Face the patient at the same level	Allows maximum interpretation of facial expression and lip movement
Ensure the patient is aware you are going to communicate	This raises the patient's attention and prepares the patient to concentrate, if necessary
Speak at a normal volume	Shouting can cause distortion of sounds. Shouting can be interpreted as aggression. Certain frequencies can not be picked up, irrespective of volume
Speak clearly but do not over pronounce lip movements	The patient may use normal lip movement as additional cues to what is being said

Action	Rationale
The speaker should not cover their mouth or turn away from the patient while speaking	The lack of visual cues may impair the patient's ability to hear
Ensure that non-verbal communication matches the content of the spoken conversation	Adds to the overall supporting cues for communication
Ensure that the patient has understood what has been said	Provides the opportunity to rephrase what has been discussed if there is no evidence of patient understanding
Consider alternative communication methods, e.g. written information if the patient continues to have difficulty understanding or is showing signs of tiredness	Patients get easily tired when concentrating on conversation. Alternative methods can reduce anxiety. Important information such as clinical procedures or medication issues should be clearly understood
Assess whether further specialist referral may be required	Patients may require further assessment/interventions
Document any difficulties and any interventions that are required/ have been carried out	Provides continuity of care and raises awareness of a hearing difficulty among healthcare staff

Procedure: Ear examination

Nurses undertaking the clinical skill of ear examination must have had the education and training stipulated by local clinical policy (Action on ENT Steering Board, 2007). Before careful physical examination of the ear, listen to the patient, elicit symptoms and take a careful history (see 'Assessment/screening questions' section above).

Equipment

- Seat/stool × 2.
- Auriscope and different sized specula.

Action	Rationale
Explain each step of any procedure or examination to the patient and gain their consent	Ensures the patient understands the process and encourages their cooperation
Decontaminate hands	
Sit the patient and self on seats at the same level	Improves access and visibility during the procedure
Examine skin of the ear, behind the ear and adjacent scalp for:	To assess the existence of any conditions
• surgery incision scars.	
• infection discharge.	
• swelling.	
• signs of skin lesions.	
• signs of skin disease.	
Do not proceed with further examination if there are signs of trauma or disease. Refer to the appropriate healthcare professional	
Use clinical judgement to select appropriately sized speculum and attach to the auriscope.	Ensures comfortable fit and optimum examination opportunity
Gently pull the pinna upwards and outwards[a]	Straightens the ear canal and maximises view
Do not continue if the patient complains of pain at this point	Localised infection or inflammation will cause this procedure to be painful
Hold the auriscope like a pen and rest the small digit (finger) on the patients' head	Digit acts as a trigger for any unexpected head movement. Reduces the risk of trauma
Switch on the auriscope light and observe the direction of the ear canal and the tympanic membrane	Avoids accidental injury from inaccurate insertion
Insert the speculum gently into the meatus to pass through the hairs at the entrance to the canal and observe through the auriscope	
Check the ear canal, tympanic membrane and mastoid cavity moving auriscope and head to ensure all is viewed	The ear cannot be assessed as normal until all the areas of the membrane are viewed. Reduces the risk of missing a condition. **It may not be possible to view the complete mastoid cavity if there has been prior surgery**

Action	Rationale
If the ability to view all of the tympanic membrane is hampered by the presence of wax, then wax removal may have to be carried out as a separate clinical procedure	
Carefully check the condition of the skin in the ear canal as you withdraw the auriscope	
Adjust seating. Select a clean speculum and repeat for the other ear	Ensures comfort during examination. Reduces cross-infection between ears
On completion of examination, return the patient to a chair of choice. Ensure that the patient is comfortable	
Clean the specula and auriscope according to patient's infection status and local infection control policy	
Decontaminate hands	
Document the procedure, ear condition, interventions/referrals required, treatment given	Individualises care
If any abnormality is detected during the examination, refer according to local policy	

(*Source:* Neno, 2006; Action on ENT Steering Board, 2007)
[a]Gently pull the pinna down and backwards in children.

HEARING AIDS

It is a myth that wearing a hearing aid will increase deafness or that tinnitus cannot be improved through use of an aid. The hissing, ringing or other associated noises may reduce with a hearing aid.

Hearing aids amplify sounds but cannot restore natural hearing (Brooker & Waugh, 2007). Therefore, hearing aids don't always return a person's hearing ability to normal and it may still be difficult to follow what people are saying in noisy places, including wards. Some hearing aids reduce certain background noises.

Hearing aids are available in different shapes, sizes and types depending at times on the disease process underpinning hearing loss. Depending on how sounds are processed, hearing aids are known as either analogue or digital. All hearing aids issued by the NHS up to the year 2000 were analogue aids (Royal National Institute for Deaf People, 2009b). Between, 2000 and 2005, the hearing aid and audiology services were 'modernised'. This included the provision of digital hearing aids, which became available to all patients in 2005. Hearing aids are becoming more sophisticated and can resolve a range of hearing problems; however, this sophistication can make understanding the controls difficult for some people (Dreschler *et al.*, 2008).

Both types of aid look very similar and it is important that the nurse knows the difference in order to help the patient maximise the benefits of using an aid.

Analogue hearing aids work through increasing the volume using a control. There is a limited ability to boost sounds of different frequencies. These hearing aids amplify all sounds in the environment indiscriminately. Consequently, in a noisy environment, the aid will amplify the noise still further. The hearing aid user is required to reduce the volume for the noise to be tolerable, which can mean that conversation is then difficult to follow. Conversely, when sounds are very soft, the aid will rely on the user to increase the volume to suit the circumstances.

Most users of analogue aids find that they continually need to adjust the volume of the hearing aid in order for the aid to be comfortable and effective. The manipulation of the controls may be difficult or even impossible for a person with a learning disability or with poor dexterity. If the adjustments cannot be made, then the user will, at times, be overpowered by too much sound, and at other times sounds will not be loud enough. This discomfort frequently leads to the aid becoming intolerable and it is consequently rejected. Up to a quarter of people who are issued with a hearing aid do not use it (Bridgewood, 2000).

Digital aids contain a processor similar to a tiny computer. The hearing test result is programmed into the aid, enabling the aid to know exactly what a person can and cannot hear. The aid then breaks down sound and amplifies it precisely according to the person's requirements. The resulting sound produced by the aid is much clearer (Royal National Institute for Deaf People, 2009b). Most digital aids can be programmed to adjust themselves automatically to suit different sound environments. They will recognise noisy and quiet environments and amplify them accordingly. This removes the need for continual adjustment and makes the aid more comfortable to wear. There is also less likely to be acoustic feedback (whistling) from the aid.

Preventing problems with hearing aids

Acoustic feedback is common and caused when amplified sound leaks out before being picked up by the microphone in the hearing aid. This squeal, whistle or buzz is caused by a poorly fitting ear mould or a mould that has not been pushed far enough into the ear. This is common as carers are often reluctant to force the ear mould into the ear. Excess wax present in the ears can also interfere with the aid, as can a damaged/ill-fitting aid, tube or mould. If the problem is not obvious or easily addressed by nursing staff, refer to the audiology department as soon as possible.

Hearing aid batteries need to be replaced every two to 12 weeks (depending on use). A hearing aid will not work with a flat battery. Regular assistance may be needed to check and change the battery. It is a good idea to stock spare batteries in the clinical area if local policy permits. This allows batteries to be available, for example, to new patients admitted outwith clinical hours. The need for a battery change is usually signalled by fainter noise through the aid or crackly, fuzzy or distorted noise. Some aids give a warning signal (a bleeping or fluttering sound) just before the battery runs flat.

Clinical staff and patients should be encouraged to store spare batteries safely, as children can swallow them or insert them into orifices such as the nose or, indeed, the ears. To ensure that the hearing aid functions as required and to reduce the number of repairs, it is important that hearing aids are maintained and cleaned regularly. It is important to establish a routine of keeping the aid in a box to protect it and to ensure it is not lost.

Different types of hearing aids and their general care
Behind-the-ear (BTE) hearing aids

These aids have an ear mould that fits snugly inside the ear. The battery-operated aid is attached to the mould by a plastic tube. The tube length is cut to allow the aid to rest behind the ear comfortably. Some models have twin microphones allowing either all-round sound or a more directional setting that lessens background disruption in noisy places. This model can also be adapted to be worn with spectacles (Department of Health, 2008).

Most BTE aids have a control switch which can indicate the status of the aid (Royal National Institute for Deaf People, 2009b):

- O: signifies that the aid is switched off.
- M: indicates that the aid is switched on and sound will be amplified.
- T: will function in places where an induction loop system is installed. This system allows the person to pick up radio signals without also picking up distorted background noise.

BTE aids should ideally have the ear mould and tubing washed daily (see 'Washing the ear mould' procedure) but at least once weekly. The hearing aid (the functioning part separate from the ear mould and tubing) should never have any liquid solution introduced (e.g. cleaning solutions) as this part is easily damaged.

Tubing connecting the hearing aid to the ear mould should be changed at least every six months. The ear mould tubing may block at intervals depending on the patient's condition and normal hygiene routines. Moisture may inadvertently be introduced or the tube (which is normally flexible) may, with age, become rigid. In any of these circumstances, the tubing will need to be replaced (see 'Washing the ear mould' procedure). The ear mould channels sound from the aid into the ear. Poor fit can affect the quality of hearing as well as the patient's comfort (Department of Health, 2008).

Insertion of the ear mould includes the following steps:

- Hold the back of the mould between finger and thumb.
- From behind the ear, lower the part of the mould that sits in the ear canal into position.
- Position the remainder of the mould into the ear.
- Using the other hand, pull the ear lobe slightly downwards and gently push the mould into the ear.
- Place the tube and aid comfortable behind the ear.

If the patient complains of discomfort or there are signs of trauma to the skin/ear through the aid being worn, then a referral to the audiologist should be made.

In-the-ear (ITE) hearing aids

ITE hearing aids (Figure 4.2) fit entirely into the ear but are not suitable for people with severe hearing loss (Brooker & Waugh, 2007). The working parts are either in a small compartment clipped to the ear mould or inside the moulded part itself. ITE aids tend to need repairing more often than BTE aids.

The entire aid should be cleaned with a dry cloth. Make sure that it does not come into contact with any liquid. Owing to the whole aid being fitted in the ear, the opening is more prone than BTE aids are to becoming blocked with wax. Often the aid comes with a wax pick, which is a small piece of equipment for removing wax from the opening at the end of the hearing aid. Substitutes for cleaning wax should be avoided to prevent damage to the aid.

Completely-in-the-canal (CIC) hearing aids

CIC hearing aids (Figure 4.3) are even smaller than ITE aids and less visible. They are unlikely to be suitable for everybody, especially those with severe hearing loss.

Body-worn hearing aids

These have a small box that can be attached to clothing or worn in a pocket. A lead connects the earphone to the box. These can be useful for people who have problems with dexterity or poor sight, as the controls tend to be larger than those of smaller aids

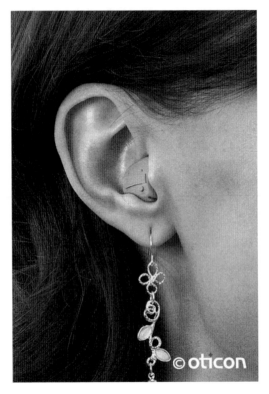

Figure 4.2 In-the-ear (ITE) hearing aid. © Oticon Ltd. Reproduced with permission.

are. Some body-worn aids are very powerful and are useful for compensating severe hearing loss. The leads of these aids often require replacing and can become damaged through becoming twisted, pulled or tangled.

Bone-conduction hearing aids

These are for people with conductive hearing loss or people who cannot wear a conventional hearing aid. They deliver sound through the skull via vibrations.

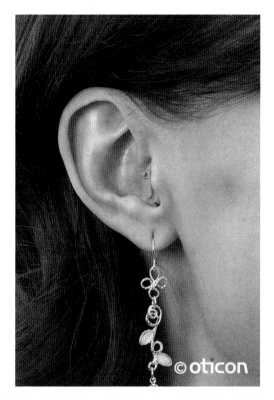

Figure 4.3 Completely-in-the-canal (CIC) hearing aid. © Oticon Ltd. Reproduced with permission.

CROS/BiCROS hearing aids

These are for people with hearing in one ear only. CROS hearing aids pick up sound from the side with no hearing and feed it to the ear with normal or near-normal hearing. BiCROS aids are similar but made for people with no useful hearing in one ear and some hearing loss in the other, so they make the sounds louder as well.

Box 4.7 Considerations for healthcare professionals when supplying a person with a hearing aid

- Does the patient have the sight and dexterity to safely insert the ear mould and switch the aid on?
- Can the patient remove the aid? If the aid becomes intolerable for any reason, would the patient be able to remove it?
- Can the user maintain the hearing aid in working order, including changing the batteries?
- Can the aid be kept safely?
- What teaching interventions and written reminders could help users and/or carers? Support may need to be arranged.

Disposable hearing aids

These are usually suitable for people with mild to moderate hearing loss. They can be thrown away and replaced when the battery runs out, which is usually after about 10 weeks.

It is important to remember that, as well as listening, most people find it helpful to watch people's faces and lip-read when in conversation. Most people lip-read in certain circumstances, for example in noisy social situations where it is difficult to be heard. Gestures and expressions are an important part of communicating, and patients may rely more on reading a nurse's body language and gestures even when using a hearing aid.

Irrespective of which type of hearing aid a person uses, their hearing problems will not be addressed if they do not have the ability or knowledge to maintain it and keep it functioning (Box 4.7). Without adequate support from healthcare staff and audiology departments, some people will not get optimum benefit from using a hearing aid (Tolson & Nolan, 2000).

MAINTENANCE OF A BEHIND-THE-EAR HEARING AID
Procedure: Washing the ear mould
Equipment

- Clean absorbent disposable drapes.
- Bowl of warm soapy water.
- Flat surface.
- Disposable wipes.

NB: This is a clean procedure and local infection control policies should be followed.

Action	Rationale
Explain each step of any procedure or examination to the patient and gain their consent	Ensures the patient understands the process and encourages their cooperation
Prepare a clean flat surface with a bowl of warm soapy water	
Decontaminate hands	
Switch off hearing aid	Reduces feedback on movement of the aid. Preserves the battery from unintentional use
Gently remove aid from ear by removing the aid and tubing from behind the ear and then gently easing the mould from the ear	Avoids potential injury to the ear. Reduces anxiety
Observe the patient's ear for redness/inflammation or any noticeable disorders	Ear moulds can cause local irritation in the ear. The tubing and aid can cause friction or irritation around the ear
Disconnect the tubing from the hearing aid. Keep the tubing in the mould	Prevents loosening of the tubing and reduction in the aid's efficiency
Lay the hearing aid on a clean drape away from risk of splashing	Reduces the risk of water damage to the aid
Wash the ear mould in warm soapy water, including the tubing	Prevents blocking of the tubing and reduction in hearing
Rinse in clear warm water	Prevents irritation to the skin from soap
Check that the tubing is not twisted, split or squashed	Prevents poor sound transmission from the aid. Twisted or split tubing can irritate behind the ear
Allow the mould and tubing to dry out completely on an absorbent drape	Prevents moisture entering the hearing aid and causing damage
Wipe the aid with a dry cloth if required	The aid will have dust and debris removed, reducing the risk of irritation/infection
Reattach tubing to the hearing aid, checking for fit	Ensures optimal hearing for the patient
Return ear mould to patient's ear, ensuring a snug fit	Reduces the risk of irritation or reduced efficiency. Reduces acoustic feedback through a poor fit

Continued

Action	Rationale
Fit tubing and aid around ear, ensuring that the tube is not too loose/tight	Reduces the risk of friction to the skin and increases the aid's efficiency
Switch on and check with the patient that aid settings are correct	Reduces the risk of whistling/acoustic feedback
OR	Keeps the aid clean and reduces the risk of damage whilst not in use
Return hearing aid to storage box until required by the patient	
Decontaminate hands	
Document interventions and evaluations of care	
Identify any referral required	

Procedure: Retubing the ear mould
Equipment

- A clean flat surface or a flat surface with a clean drape.
- Tubing.
- Sterile scissors.

NB: This is a clean procedure and local infection control policies should be followed.

Action	Rationale
Explain each step of any procedure or examination to the patient and gain their consent	Ensures the patient understands the process and encourages their cooperation
Decontaminate hands	
Detach the mould from the hearing aid	
Pull out the old piece of tube from the mould and keep it	Provides a template for the replacement tubing
Cut one end of a new piece of tubing to a point	Allows ease of movement through the ear mould
Push the pointed end through the hole on the back of the mould (the flat side) allowing the tube to bend upwards	Allows optimum fit when returned to the ear

Action	Rationale
Pull the tube all the way through the mould until you reach the bend in the tubing and the uncut end faces upright	Facilitates measuring for individual requirements and fit
Cut the pointed end of the tube flush with the tip of the mould	Any protruding tube can make the ear sore
Using the used tubing as a template, measure the replacement tubing for fit and cut to required length	Ensures that the tube will meet individual needs and that hear aid will fit
Re-attach mould and tubing to the hearing aid, ensuring correct fit and that tubing is not twisted or cracked	Correctly fitted tubing prevents damage to the aid through separating and dropping. Increases efficiency of the aid
Return ear mould to patient's ear, ensuring a snug fit	Reduces the risk of irritation or reduced efficiency
Fit tubing and aid around ear, ensuring that the tube is not too loose/tight	Reduces the risk of friction to the skin and increases the aid's efficiency
Switch on and check with the patient that aid settings are correct OR Return hearing aid to storage box until required by the patient	Reduces the risk of whistling/ feedback Keeps the aid clean and reduces the risk of damage whilst not in use

(*Source:* Kelleher & Moulding, 2009)

CONCLUSION

This chapter has highlighted that communication difficulties through hearing impairment impact on physical, psychological and social health. People with hearing problems may find themselves isolated and/or depressed with limited access to help or resources. Hearing problems can severely limit participation in activities and contribute to an increased risk of falls and accidents.

Poor nursing assessment and lack of referral to specialist healthcare staff have the potential to reduce quality of life for people with hearing loss. Sensitive and responsive nursing care can improve patients' confidence and ability to cope with hearing and ear problems.

APPENDIX 4.1

Screening version of the Hearing Handicap Inventory for the Elderly (HHIE-S)

Item	Yes (4 pts)	Sometimes (2 pts)	No (0 pts)
Does a hearing problem cause you to feel embarrassed when you meet new people?			
Does a hearing problem cause you to feel frustrated when talking to members of your family?			
Do you have difficulty hearing when someone speaks in a whisper?			
Do you feel handicapped by a hearing problem?			
Does a hearing problem cause you difficulty when visiting friends, relatives, or neighbours?			
Does a hearing problem cause you to attend religious services less often than you would like?			
Does a hearing problem cause you to have arguments with family members?			
Does a hearing problem cause you difficulty when listening to TV or radio?			
Do you feel that any difficulty with your hearing limits or hampers your personal or social life?			
Does a hearing problem cause you difficulty when in a restaurant with relatives or friends?			

Raw score _____ (sum of the points assigned to each of the items)
Interpreting the raw score
0–8 = 13% probability of hearing impairment (no handicap/no referral)
10–24 = 50% probability of hearing impairment (mild–moderate handicap/refer)
26–40 = 84% probability of hearing impairment (severe handicap/refer)
Referral for a score of >10 (Demers, 2004)

(*Source:* Reuben DB, Walsh EK, Moore AA, Damesyn M, Greendale GA (1998) Hearing loss in community-dwelling older persons: National prevalence data and identification using simple questions. *Journal of the American Geriatrics Society* **46**(8): 1008–1011. Copyright Wiley-Blackwell. Reproduced with permission.)

REFERENCES

Action on ENT Steering Board (2007) Guidance in ear care, http://www.entnursing.com/earcare.htm, [accessed 3 March 2009].

Ahmad W, Darr A, Jones L *et al.* (1998) *Deaf People from Minority Ethnic Groups: Initiatives and Services.* Joseph Rowntree Foundation, York.

Aung T, Mulley GP (2002) 10-minute consultation: removal of ear wax. *British Medical Journal* **325**: 27, http://www.bmj.com/cgi/content/full/325/7354/27 [accessed 11 December 2009].

Baer S (2005) Knowing when to treat ear wax. *Practitioner* **11**: 328.

Bagai A, Thavendiranathan P, Detsky AS (2006) Does this patient have hearing impairment? *Journal of the American Medical Association* **295**(4): 416–428.

Block SL (2005) Otitis externa: Providing relief while avoiding complications. *Journal of Family Practice* **54**(8): 669–676.

Bluestone CD (2000) Clinical course, complications and sequelae of acute otitis media. *Pediatric Infectious Disease Journal* **19**(5): (supplement): S37–S46.

Bridgewood A (2000) *People Aged 65 and Over: General Household survey.* Office of National Statistics, London.

British Tinnitus Association (2000) The nurse's role in helping people with tinnitus, http://www.tinnitus.org.uk/index.php?q=node/73, [accessed 3 March 2009].

Brooker C, Waugh A (2007) *Foundations of Nursing Practice: Fundamentals of holistic care.* Elsevier, London.

Browning G (2004) Ear wax. *Clinical Evidence* **12**: 730–741.

BUPA (2008) Middle ear infection in children, http://hcd2.bupa.co.uk/fact_sheets/mosby_factsheets/otitis_media.html, [accessed 20 October 2009].

Burton MJ, Doree CJ (2003) *Ear Drops for the Removal of Ear Wax (Cochrane Review).* The Cochrane Library, Issue 3, John Wiley & Sons, Ltd, London, http://www.thecochranelibrary.com, [accessed 1 March 2009].

Chamley CA, Carson P, Randall D et al. (2005) *Developmental Anatomy and Physiology of Children.* Elsevier, London.

Cook KA, Walsh M (2005) Otitis media, http://www.emedicine.com, [accessed 3 March 2009].

Corker M (1998) *Deaf and Disabled or Deaf Disabled?* Open University Press, Buckingham.

Daugherty J (2007) The latest buzz on tinnitus. *Nurse Practitioner* **32**(10): 42–47.

Demers K (2004) Try this: Best practices in nursing care to older adults: *Hearing screening*. Dermatology Nursing **16**(2): 199–200.

Department of Health (2008) *How to Use Your Hearing Aid*. DH, London.

Dreschler WA, Keidser G, Convery E *et al.* (2008) Client-based adjustments of hearing aid gain: The effect of different control configurations. *Ear and Hearing* **29**(2): 214–227.

Fligor BJ, Cox LC (2004) Output levels of commercially available portable disc players and the potential risk to hearing. *Ear and Hearing* **25**(6): 513–517.

Gates GA, Murphy M, Rees TS, Fraher A (2003) Screening for handicapping hearing loss in the elderly. *Journal of Family Practice* **52**(1): 56–62.

Hand C, Harvey I (2004) The effectiveness of topical preparations for the treatment of earwax: A systematic review. *British Journal of General Practice* **54**(508): 862–867.

Harkin H (2005) *Procedure for Ear Irrigation (and Instrumentation)*. Procedure number 68. Rotherham NHS Primary Care Trust on behalf of the Action on ENT Steering Group.

Kelleher C, Moulding L (2009) Communicating with patients who are hard of hearing or deaf, http://www.entnursing.com/nursesleaflet.htm, [accessed 3 March 2009].

Ménière's Society (2009) About Ménière's disease: How it affects you, http://www.menieres.org.uk/about_md_how_it_affects_you.html, [accessed 3 March 2009].

Mills L (2008) Management of otitis media. *Nurse Prescribing* **6**(5): 197–200.

National Institute for Occupational Safety and Health (1996) Preventing occupational hearing loss: A practical guide, http://www.cdc.gov/niosh/docs/96-110/default.html, [accessed 3 March 2009].

Neno R (2006) Holistic ear care: Cerumen removal techniques. *Journal of Community Nursing* **20**(9): 26–30.

NHS Quality Improvement Scotland (2005) *Maximising communication with older people who have hearing disability*. NHS QIS, Edinburgh.

NHS Quality Improvement Scotland (2006) *Best Practice Statement: Ear care*. NHS QIS, Edinburgh.

NHS Scotland (2005) ENT: Aural discharge patient pathway (adults), http://www.pathways.scot.nhs.uk, [accessed 3 March 2009].

Nursing and Midwifery Council (2008) *Standards for Medicines Management*. NMC, London.

Osbourne GO (2009) About Meniere's disease, http://www.menieres. org.uk/about_menieres_disease.html, [accessed 3 March 2009].

Rees T (2004) Hearing loss: Causes, symptoms and communication. *Nursing and Residential Care* **6**(1): 13–16.

Rodgers R (2003) Primary ear care treatments. *Practice Nurse* **25**(9): 6973.

Roeser RJ, Ballachanda BB (1997) Physiology, pathophysiology and anthropology/epidemiology of human ear canal secretions. *Journal of the American Academy of Audiology* **8**(6): 391–400.

Roland PS, Smith TL, Schwartz SR (2008) Clinical practice guideline: Cerumen impaction. *Otolaryngology: Head and Neck Surgery* **139**(3) (suppl. 2): S1–S21.

Royal College of Paediatrics and Child Health (2003) *Medicines for Children*. Royal College of Paediatrics and Child Health, London.

Royal National Institute for Deaf People (2004) Deaf and hard of hearing people, http://www.rnid.org.uk/information_resources/factsheets/ deaf_awareness/factsheets_leaflets/deaf_and_hard_of_hearing_ people.htm, [accessed 10 October 2009].

Royal National Institute for Deaf People (2007) About deafness and hearing loss: Members' survey, http://www.RNID.org/survey, [accessed 3 March 2009].

Royal National Institute for Deaf People (2009a) Members' survey, http://www.rnid.org.uk/information_resources/aboutdeafness/sta- tistics/member_survey/, [accessed 22 October 2009].

Royal National Institute for Deaf People (2009b) *Caring for Older People Who Have a Hearing Loss*. RNID, London.

Royal National Institute for Deaf People (2009c) Types of hearing loss – conductive and sensorineural, http://www.rnid.org.uk/information_ resources/aboutdeafness/causes/conductive_sensorineural_hearing_ loss/, [accessed 22 October 2009].

Sander R (2001) Otitis externa: A practical guide to treatment and preven- tion. *American Family Physician* **63**(5): 927–936.

Scottish Council on Deafness (2009) *Access to Information: Position State- ment*. SCD, Glasgow.

SIGN (2003) *Diagnosis and Management of Childhood Otitis Media in Primary Care*. SIGN, Edinburgh.

Somerville G (2002) The most effective products available to facilitate ear syringing. *British Journal of Community Nursing* **7**(2): 94– 101.

Stevens D (2008) Earache. *Practice Nursing* **19**(4), 193–195.

Thibodeau GA, Patton KT (2008) *Structure and Function of the Body*, 13th edn. Mosby Elsevier, St Louis.

Tolson D, Nolan M (2000) Gerontological nursing 4: Age-related hearing explored. *British Journal of Nursing* **9**(4): 205–208.

Tolson D, Swan I, Knussen C (2002) Hearing disability: A source of distress for older people and carers. *British Journal of Nursing* **11**(15): 1021–1025.

Wallhagen MI, Pettengill E, Whiteside M (2006) Sensory impairment in older adults: Part 1: Hearing loss. *American Journal of Nursing* **106**(10): 40–48.

Warrell DA, Cox TM, Firth JD (eds) (2003) *Oxford Textbook of Medicine. Volume 3*, 4th edn. Oxford University Press, New York.

Waugh A, Grant A (2004) *Ross and Wilson Anatomy and Physiology in Health and Illness*, 9th edn. Churchill Livingstone, Edinburgh.

Williamson I, Benge S, Mullee M *et al.* (2006) Consultations for middle ear disease, antibiotic prescribing and risk factors for reattendance: A case-linked cohort study. *British Journal of General Practice* **56**(524): 170–175.

Yardley L (1994) *Vertigo and Dizziness*. Routledge Press, London.

Yardley L, Beech S, Zander L *et al.* (1998) A randomized controlled trial of exercise therapy for dizziness and vertigo in primary care. *British Journal of General Practice* **48**(429): 1136–1140.

Foot and Nail Care

5

THE IMPORTANCE OF FOOT AND NAIL CARE

Mobility is an important activity of living, particularly when considering independence in self-care. Being able to mobilise lessens the length of time people stay in hospital; the risks of falling and developing pressure sores are similarly reduced. If the patient feels unbalanced when walking, has discomfort or pain or if their gait is abnormal when walking due to painful feet or foot conditions, they are less likely to want to mobilise, or to mobilise effectively. Foot pain has been found to impair functional ability more than any other single foot condition (Menz & Lord, 2001a), but the cumulative effect of multiple foot problems has more influence over falls than the presence or absence of individual foot conditions (Menz & Lord, 2001b). Foot and nail care therefore is fundamental to mobility, comfort and independence (Bryant & Beinlich, 1999).

The aim of this chapter is to help the reader understand how to carry out fingernail care, toenail care and the underpinning rationale(s) for foot care.

LEARNING OUTCOMES

After reading this chapter, the reader will be able to:

❏ Understand the impact of poor foot health on mobility.
❏ Identify common conditions during assessment.
❏ Assess for factors impacting on mobility.
❏ Describe the anatomy and physiology of finger- and toenails.
❏ Understand and carry out clinical care of the patient's fingernails.
❏ Understand and carry out clinical care of the patient's toenails.

❏ Understand the evidence base underpinning clinical procedures.

Almost half of people over 75 say better foot care would improve their health and quality of life; disabled people identify podiatrists as the most important NHS service after GPs (George, 1995). However, over the past 10–15 years, there has been a reorganisation of services and nurses have been expected to take over some of the less complex foot care, such as toenail cutting and foot care (Department of Health, 1994). It has been suggested that nurses lack the skills, education and equipment to carry out foot care and traditionally depend on podiatrists to carry out these activities (George, 1995). However, incorporating robust foot care interventions improves the patient's care overall and complies with the *Essence of Care* benchmarking (Department of Health, 2001), which identifies that all hygiene needs should be met.

THE INFLUENCE OF LIFESPAN ON FOOT HEALTH AND HYGIENE

Infancy (0–23 months)

The bones have not been fully formed in the limbs or feet after birth, although ossification (bone formation) begins in the embryonic stage. The bones of the ankle and heel (tarsus) are formed by birth but the foot does not completely mature until the age of 5 years (Chamley *et al.*, 2005). A newborn's ankles are very supple, but the foot itself is very chubby and the foot appears flat. Shoes only protect the feet at this age and don't help a baby to stand or walk; therefore, they are not required until a baby is standing and attempting to walk. A 1-year-old will outgrow shoes every 1–2 months and will require larger socks.

Congenital abnormalities of the limbs occur in approximately 1–2:1000 live births (Chamley *et al.*, 2005), ranging from major deformities in development to the relatively minor (but not necessarily to the child or its parents) deficits or alteration of digits (toes). Talipes equinovarus (club foot), where the foot is axially rotated outwards but points inwards, is one of the more commonly known congenital conditions. The condition may be in isolation or associated with other disorders such as spina bifida.

Childhood (2–12 years)

The metatarsal bones (one of the five cylindrical bones extending from the heel (the tarsus) to the toes on each foot) are formed, but are not fixed at this age. Poorly fitting shoes at this age can lead to chronic foot problems in adulthood. Shoes should be straight when looked at from beneath and a good fit. Children should have their feet measured about every three months and there should be a thumb width between the end of the shoe and the end of the longest toe (Thomson *et al.*, 2001). Foot disorders rarely occur during childhood, as even the effects of poorly fitting shoes are not evident until later in life (Frey, 2000).

Adolescence (13–19 years)

Hands and feet grow more rapidly than the rest of the skeleton during the onset of puberty (Chamley *et al.*, 2005) but stop growing before the rest of the skeleton. The metatarsal bones fuse by the age of 18 years. At this age, the most common foot condition is athlete's foot (tinea pedis), and teenagers should be given advice about foot hygiene and particularly about care of trainers and footwear.

Nail health can be influenced by diet in this age group. Teenagers with eating disorders or those who fail to achieve a balanced diet may develop brittle nails (Scher *et al.*, 2003).

Adulthood (20–64 years)

Women have a higher incidence of foot problems than men do (Frey, 2000). The causes are mostly attributable to poor-fitting footwear the wearing of shoes that are primarily fashionable rather than comfortable. Footwear has changed from the soft, flexible moccasins of early humans to the rigid, fashion footwear that is available currently. Poorly fitting shoes can gradually remould the foot, pushing small toes inward and sometimes over other toes (Bryant & Beinlich, 1999). The result of this is a high prevalence of conditions such as corns, calluses, bunions and hammer toes (Dickson *et al.*, 2008). A woman between 50 and 60 years of age can count on her foot being larger than it was when she was in her twenties and she should wear the appropriate shoe size (Menz & Lord, 2001b). Men have fewer problems because of the nature of their shoes (i.e. flatter and wider). Nail appearance changes as early as the late twenties, where nails begin to develop longitudinal ridges and become less flexible (Scher *et al.*, 2003). Conditions which develop in adulthood may influence nail health, for example anaemia, endocrine disorders and pregnancy can all result in brittle or splitting nails.

Older age (65+ years)

Between 50 and 70% of older people report foot problems (Menz & Lord, 2001b). Natural ageing changes can affect an older person's balance (e.g. there is a decrease in bone mass and muscle tone). Older people are more likely to suffer a range of medical conditions which affect foot health, for example diabetes, arthritic changes and diseases of the nervous system that can affect a person's sensation in the feet (Badlissi *et al.*, 2005). Normal circulatory changes with ageing also render the skin more easily damaged, and healing times take longer. Reduced sight and dexterity of the fingers can contribute to difficulty for an older person to maintain good foot hygiene and short toenails. They may wear ill-fitting shoes for the sake of ease. This compromises safety; in one study, 28% of older people who were investigated for falling stated that the shoe was the primary cause (Menz & Lord, 2001b). Toenails become thicker and more brittle with age. Reduced flexibility and joint problems may mean that older people have difficulty cutting their toenails. Long nails may grow towards the back of the toes, causing pressure and reducing the ability to mobilise without pain. Narrowing of the blood vessels means that nails will become more brittle.

PHYSICAL INFLUENCES ON FOOT HEALTH AND FOOT HYGIENE

Older people may have reduced circulation or nerve damage, resulting in the loss of feeling or altered sensation in their feet. If this is the case, to avoid the effects of accidental damage to the feet and delayed healing, nurses should refer toenail care to the podiatrist.

Aside from ageing, the most common risk to healthy feet comes from the condition diabetes mellitus. Around two million people in the UK are known to have diabetes and many more are thought to be undiagnosed (Diabetes UK, 2004).

Diabetes mellitis is usually characterised by a person having too high a level of sugar (glucose) in the blood. The most common forms of diabetes are type 1 and type 2.

Type 1 is caused by the body's failure to produce the hormone insulin. Insulin is released by the pancreas to help control levels of sugar in the blood. Type 1 usually appears before the age of 40 and is referred to as 'juvenile' or 'early onset' diabetes. Type 1 is usually more detectable than type 2 (American Diabetes Association, 2008).

Type 2 is caused by the body not producing enough insulin or not effectively using the insulin produced. This is the more common form and accounts for around 90% of all cases of diabetes (Diabetes UK, 2004). Unfortunately, owing to the often vague symptoms of diabetes type 2, many people are unaware that they have the condition until complications from the disease arise, such as wounds on the feet that are slow to heal (Fletcher, 2006).

Hyperglycaemia (high blood sugar) can harm the blood vessels that carry oxygen and nutrients to the nerves (Diabetes UK, 2008). These structural changes mean that a person with diabetes may develop nerve damage (neuropathy), where their feet may feel numb or tingly. This nerve damage along with vascular insufficiency (poor circulation), infection and pressure on the foot predispose the person with diabetes to develop foot ulceration (Baker *et al.*, 2005a, 2005b).

Five to fifteen per cent of people with diabetes will develop a foot ulcer at some point (National Institute for Health and Clinical Excellence, 2008), which if poorly treated can lead to amputation (Diabetes UK, 2004).

PSYCHOLOGICAL INFLUENCES ON FOOT HEALTH AND FOOT HYGIENE

Some women, and more so than men, may put up with pain or discomfort in order to wear shoes that are more stylish, or make them feel more sexually alluring, than are comfortable. Many people – again more women than men – choose not to wear corrective footwear, which may have been prescribed for them (Williams *et al.*, 2008). This is commonly because there is a perception that the footwear is unattractive.

However, having unattractive feet also causes psychological distress and some people are embarrassed at showing their feet, even to healthcare professionals. Sensitivity is important when offering advice to patients and when carrying out nursing interventions.

SOCIOCULTURAL INFLUENCES ON FOOT HEALTH AND FOOT HYGIENE

Type 2 diabetes, referred to as 'the silent assassin', has reached pandemic proportions worldwide (Diabetes UK, 2008). A million amputations are carried out annually as a direct result of poor diabetes care. The main causes behind the increasing numbers of diabetics are linked to rapid cultural changes, ageing populations, increasing urbanisation, dietary changes, decreased physical activity and other unhealthy lifestyles. In the UK, people who originate from Africa and southern Asia have shown a dramatic rise in the incidence of Type 2 diabetes. Some older people, and particularly women, who do not have English as their first language are likely to be undiagnosed.

ENVIRONMENTAL INFLUENCES ON FOOT HEALTH AND FOOT HYGIENE

It is clear that footwear influences foot health; babies and children have few conditions which are not congenital and foot health declines as we get older in direct relation to the shoes we choose to wear. Nurses can give patients advice about footwear as a health promotion and educational strategy (Box 5.1).

POLITICO-ECONOMIC INFLUENCES ON FOOT HEALTH AND FOOT HYGIENE

There is currently an average of one podiatrist to over 2000 older people. Increasing demand for podiatry services has led to ration-

---

Box 5.1 Advice about footwear

- Shoes should be comfortable, well-fitting and supportive.
- Shoes should accommodate the toes without altering their shape or cramping them.
- Slippers should not be worn for long periods as they do not provide sufficient support and cause poor posture and a shuffling gait.
- Shoe material should be able to breathe; avoid synthetic materials.
- Low-heeled shoes with non-slip soles are advisable for long-term wear to increase stability.
- Keep the wearing of fashion shoes to a minimum.
- Shoes should be wider than the top and front of the feet when looking down.
- Shoes should not be worn if they cause pain.

(*Source:* Bryant & Beinlich, 1999)

---

ing, with people considered low risk no longer being eligible for NHS podiatry (Department of Health, 2008). The longer-term impact of denying treatment to those considered to have a low risk is yet to be established. It has been suggested that 25% of people needing foot care are no longer eligible for NHS care (Department of Health, 2008). Although there is no direct evidence that a lack of podiatry provision for older people results in care home admissions, poor foot health can lead to social isolation, decreased mobility and an increase in the number of falls and fractures. It could be deduced that there may be a number of people who are admitted as an indirect consequence of poor foot health/care. Recognition of the problem has led to the reorganisation of services, where uncomplicated nail cutting and foot care have been separated from more skilled interventions provided by podiatry and specialist services. As a result, nurses are expected to take on a larger role than before in maintaining and improving foot health (George, 1995).

FOOT CARE

Advice about general foot care will support any guidance about footwear. This is particularly important for older people, who through the natural ageing process may be at risk of reduced circulation to the lower limbs. Patients should be encouraged to remain active within the clinical area and take short walks frequently (Fletcher, 2006). Nurses should incorporate planned walks into the patient's care plan if the patient needs assistance to mobilise. Foot exercises should be encouraged at least on a once-daily basis (see 'Foot assessment' procedure).

COMMON FOOT CONDITIONS
Arthritic feet
Arthritis is described as inflammation and swelling of the cartilage and lining of the joints, usually accompanied by an increase in the fluid in the joints. Osteoarthritis, also called degenerative joint disease, is the most common form of arthritis. It is characterised by the breakdown of cartilage in joints, which causes joint stiffness. As osteoarthritis progresses, bone spurs (osteophytes) develop within the affected joint and the joint space narrows, pain increases and mobility becomes more difficult (Badlissi *et al.*, 2005). Suitable footwear is vital for people with arthritis in order to prevent skin trauma, corns and calluses (Williams *et al.*, 2008). Footwear is likely to be prescribed as a result of referral to an orthotics specialist.

Diabetic foot ulcers
The most common location for foot ulcers is on the plantar surface of the forefoot (American Diabetes Association, 2008). A person with neuropathy may not be alerted to any trauma occurring to the foot, as they have no sensation of pain. If the foot has poor circulation, the healing of any trauma will be delayed and there will be an increased risk of infection (Edwards, 2008).

Patients may not be aware that they have diabetes until they present with a wound to the foot that is slow to heal. Nurses have been identified as not taking opportunities with patients to advise them about maintaining foot health (Brookes & O'Leary, 2006). Advice about foot care should be given as above, but additionally people with diabetes should be advised to avoid direct sources of heat (e.g. sitting with feet close to a radiator or soaking the feet in hot water). Very importantly, the patient should be advised to never walk about barefoot. Not wearing shoes causes an increased risk of accidental injury to the foot, which either may not be felt or is slow to heal. Generally, foot injuries cause people pain and to change their gait (way of walking) to compensate and avoid putting pressure on the wound (Kravitz *et al.*, 2003); people with diabetes may continue to walk as normal and the wound then becomes larger and even more difficult to heal (Mayfield *et al.*, 1998). Fluid also collects under callus (hard skin) formation and becomes infected, leading to abscesses and ulceration. The opening of the ulcer may be small and the extent of the tissue damage may not be obvious from observation (Leese *et al.*, 2007).

People with diabetes should never use over-the-counter topical preparations that remove warts or corns, because they can burn the skin and cause damage to the foot of a diabetic sufferer. Nor should they try any home treatments such as cutting calluses as trauma may occur. Any foot problems should be referred directly to the podiatrist.

In addition to assessing the risk of developing a foot ulcer from direct examination of the foot (Table 5.1), general risk factors should also be assessed and treated or advice offered (Brookes & O'Leary, 2006), including:

- Blood pressure.
- Blood sugar level and insulin use.
- Cardiovascular disease.
- Smoking.
- Alcohol.
- Weight.

Healing diabetic foot ulcers will require variable nursing interventions, all of which will support the regime identified by the podiatrist, medical specialist and tissue viability specialist. Treatment may include antibiotic therapy, surgical debridement, non-surgical interventions such as prescribed topical preparations, pressure relief of the affected area and possible modified footwear. However, antibiotics may not reach the infected wound, because of impaired blood flow, and in severe infection may be ineffective. Then often the only way to prevent septicaemia (blood poisoning) is to amputate the foot or leg (Leese *et al.*, 2007).

Table 5.1 Level of risk for developing foot ulcers

Risk level	Nursing action
Low risk: normal circulation, pulses palpable, normal sensation (feeling) in the feet	Plan care with the patient Education and advice in maintaining foot health will be required Assess foot health as part of daily care
Increased risk: evidence of neuropathy, poor or absent pulses	Refer to foot care team or podiatrist Evaluate footwear Offer advice on foot care Assess foot health as part of daily care
High risk: evidence of neuropathy, absent pulses, skin changes, history of a previous ulcer	Refer to foot care team or podiatrist Evaluate footwear Assess foot health as part of daily care Perform foot care as part of daily care
Foot ulcerated	Refer to specialist as an emergency and follow planned care accordingly Evaluate and reassess the ulcer on a daily basis

(*Source:* National Institute for Health and Clinical Excellence, 2008)

When evaluating care, a 50% reduction in wound surface area after four weeks is a good predictor of wound healing at 12 weeks (Sheehan *et al.*, 2003). However, failure to show improvement after four weeks may be an indicator of future amputation. Incomplete healing may be due to a failure to reduce the pressure on the wound through the patient continuing to mobilise.

Full healing of diabetic foot ulcers may not always be possible and the wound will become chronic. Planned outcomes may change and the patient should be involved in the process. Expected outcomes may change to reducing pain, reducing the risk of infection and finding a wound dressing regime that suits the patient (Edmonds & Foster, 2006).

Patients with neuropathic foot ulcers may be required to wear casts or footwear to redistribute plantar pressures on the ulcer and promote healing. This may be achieved by using padding in footwear, but a more effective measure is to use a total ready made prefabricated contact cast boot (Edmonds & Foster, 2006).

Fungal infections

Fungal infections of the foot are common in people of all ages and can affect either the skin (tinea pedis) or the toenails (onychomycosis) (Crawford & Hollis, 2008). The severity and duration of the infection is dependent on the area of the foot affected. The cause of the infection is most frequently a dermatophyte (fungus), which inhabits and destroys the protein keratin.

Athlete's foot (tinea pedis)

Athlete's foot is a fungal infection, causing upper layers of the skin to flake away, exposing the more sensitive deeper layers of the skin. Footwear, often the cause, creates a warm, static environment with the correct pH in which bacteria and fungi can breed. There are several different presentations of tinea pedis, which could be confused with other non-infectious skin conditions:

- Interdigital tinea pedis: the skin between the toes is macerated (wet) and scaly. Particularly affects the outer toes. The skin may crack.
- Plantar type tinea pedis (moccasin foot): presents as fine powdery scaling over redness that covers the skin of the soles, heels and sides of the foot.
- Vesicular (bullous) type: caused by an acute inflammatory condition, characterised by the presence of vesicles, pustules or blisters. This can be confused with foot dermatitis.

(Bell-Syer *et al.*, 2002)

COMMON FOOT ABNORMALITIES
Bunions

A bunion is an enlargement of the joint at the base of the big toe, the metatarsophalangeal (MTP) joint. A bunion develops when the bone or tissue at the joint moves out of place forcing the big toe to bend towards the others. The result is a lump of bone on the foot which can cause extreme pain if untreated as the body weight from walking is carried by this joint. The wearing of normal-fitting shoes may be difficult or impossible.

Box 5.2 Advice for patients regarding the treatment and management of bunions

- Initial treatment: apply a commercial, non-medicated bunion pad around the bony prominence (minimises pain and allows the patient to continue a normal, active life).
- Taping the foot maintains a normal position, reducing stress and pain.
- Shoes should have a wide and deep toe.
- If inflamed and painful, apply ice packs several times a day to reduce the swelling.
- Avoid wearing shoes with heels over two inches high.
- Refer to the podiatrist.
- Always buy shoes to fit the foot with the bunion or the larger foot.
- Anti-inflammatory drugs and cortisone injections are often prescribed to ease acute pain and inflammations.
- Shoe inserts may be useful in controlling foot function and may reduce symptoms and prevent worsening of the deformity.

(*Source:* American Podiatric Medical Association, 2009)

The primary goal of most early treatment options is to relieve pressure on the bunion and halt the progression of the joint deformity. This can be achieved in part by offering advice regarding footwear and specialist interventions (Box 5.2).

Corns (helomas) and calluses (keratomas)

These are thickened areas of skin. They are caused by repeated friction and pressure from skin rubbing against bony areas or against an irregularity in a shoe or by wearing overly tight shoes (American Podiatric Medical Association, 2009). Corns ordinarily form on the toes and are usually hard and circular, with a waxy or translucent centre. They may become painful or ulcerated in response to continued friction. Calluses are more likely to form on the soles of the feet. They form to protect the skin and the structures beneath it from injury or damage and can develop on any part of the body. Both can be painful and may be relieved by padding on the affected areas and wearing well-fitting shoes. Never cut corns or calluses with any instrument, and home remedies should be used with caution; people with circulatory problems and diabetics should not use any treatments except under a podiatrist's instructions.

NURSING ASSESSMENT OF THE FEET

The feet probably undergo the greatest stresses and strains of any part of the body; all of our body weight is carried by our feet and they constantly cope with pressure. Foot care requires a multi-disciplinary approach. There will be patients who are at a low risk of developing foot problems when nursing interventions will be adequate to maintain foot health. Other patients may be at an increased risk, which will reduce their mobility and be dangerous to their general health (Burrow, 2004). These patients will require referral to specialist healthcare professionals such as podiatrists, dermatologists, vascular surgeons and tissue viability specialists. A family history should be assessed as to whether there is any history of diabetes, circulatory/heart problems or any other condition(s) which may affect foot health. Lifestyle issues can also be assessed, for example smoking and alcohol can both contribute to poor circulation, which in turn can cause poor foot health, ulcers or chronic wounds. A physical examination of the feet and lower limbs can allow the nurse to determine any risk to foot health or establish if there are any current foot conditions which will require either specialist or nursing interventions (Box 5.3).

Procedure: Foot assessment
Equipment

- Personal protective equipment (PPE).
- Footstool (if the patient is sitting).

Box 5.3 Patient groups who should be referred to specialist services

- Any patient with a medical condition affecting their feet (e.g. diabetes or vascular disease).
- Any patient who is prescribed regular oral, intramuscular or intravenous steroids (e.g. prednisolone).
- Any patient prescribed regular anticoagulants (e.g. warfarin).
- Any patient who has foot abnormalities (e.g. corns, calluses, bunions).

(*Source:* Fletcher, 2006)

- Protective cover for the footstool.
- Prescribed care if appropriate.

Action	Rationale
Check the patient's care plan and prescription sheet for details of current foot conditions, prescribed care, planned care and nursing interventions	Allows the nurse to implement and evaluate care
Explain each step of any procedure or examination to the patient and gain their consent	Ensures the patient understands the process and encourages their cooperation
Ensure privacy	Preserves dignity. Patients may be uncomfortable exposing their feet
Using appropriate moving and handling techniques, assist the patient into a comfortable position – ideally, sitting in a chair at a height where the patient can place their feet on the floor. Alternatively, the patient should lie supine with a pillow under their knees to raise and support	Prevents muscle fatigue and allows the patient to cope with the procedure
Decontaminate hands and put on PPE; gloves can be used if there is a risk of infection or if the patient's skin is broken	Wearing an apron reduces the risk of cross-infection from the nurse's uniform
Ask the patient if they have any feelings of pain, tingling or numbness in the feet or toes	Identifies the possible presence of circulatory problems or neuropathy
Ask the patient/assist the patient to remove their footwear	Allows assessment of independence in the activity
Ask the patient to place their feet on the footstool, which has been covered with a protective sheet	
Inspect each lower leg and foot for: Swelling	Swelling may indicate poor circulation or the presence of infection

Action	Rationale
Discoloration	Pale skin denotes possible circulatory problems, black areas indicate prolonged unrelieved pressure (ischaemia), red areas indicate pressure or the presence of inflammation/infection
Skin breaks	Skin breaks indicate the presence of trauma, ulceration or pressure, ill-fitting footwear or infection (e.g. athlete's foot)
Cracks or fissures between the toes	Cracks or fissures between the toes indicate the presence of fungal infection, or dry skin, which is at risk of becoming infected
Observe the patient's toenails for:	
Discoloration of nails	Discoloration signifies the presence of infection (yellowing/brownish) or trauma (red or blackened) to the nail bed.
Abnormalities in appearance or separation of the nail from the nail bed	Abnormalities signify the presence of trauma or infection.
Debris under the nail, thickened nails, discoloured nails, musty-smelling nails, flaking of the nails	Signifies the presence of fungal infection (although thickened nails may also be attributed to normal ageing)
Brittle nails	Aside from becoming more brittle with normal ageing, poor circulation also causes brittle nails
Touching the patient's lower legs and feet:	
Check for temperature differences between both legs/feet and in comparison to other parts of the body	Warmer areas may indicate the presence of infection. Cooler areas may indicate poor circulation.
Check the firmness (turgor) of the skin on the lower legs/feet: pinch the skin gently and assess how rapidly the skin returns to normal	Skin which does not return to normal on gentle pinching may signify dehydration.
Check the texture of the skin for roughness or dry areas	Skin which is coarse or dry may be more at risk of breaking or cracking.

Continued

Action	Rationale
Observe for: • Signs of dirt or infection in the skin folds of the feet, e.g. under/ between the toes. • Evidence of self-neglect. • Signs of disease. • Signs of excessive perspiration.	These may signify that the patient has been unable to carry out self-care of their feet
If not the first assessment, evaluate the effectiveness of planned nursing interventions regarding treating or maintaining foot health	Allows the nurse to compare the current lower leg and feet condition to the baseline assessment and to determine if the patient's condition(s) is improving or deteriorating
Ask/assist the patient to perform foot exercises: circle the foot clockwise several times and repeat in an anticlockwise direction; flex the foot downwards and upwards several times	Daily (or more frequent) exercising improves the circulation to the feet, reducing swelling and the risk of pressure. Allows assessment of the patient's flexibility and ability to undertake exercises
Offer advice regarding maintaining/ improving foot health	
If foot hygiene interventions are not being carried out at this point, ask/ assist the patient to put on clean footwear. Assess whether the patient's footwear is suitable and offer advice	Allows assessment of self-care ability. Clean footwear daily, particularly cotton socks, allows the feet to breathe and reduces the risk of acquiring a fungal infection
Assist the patient into a comfortable position and check that no further care is required at this time	
Clear away any used equipment, remove PPE and decontaminate hands	Prevents cross-infection
Document the evaluation of the patient's condition and nursing interventions identified in the care plan	Individualises nursing care
Document and report any new abnormalities or any concerns the patient has	Identifies actual or potential problems with foot health
Document and report any referrals required and the time frame for reassessment	Directs patient care

Procedure: Foot hygiene
Equipment

- Basin of warm water and bath thermometer.
- Jug of warm water.
- Towels.
- Absorbent sheet, e.g. disposable pad.
- PPE.
- Topical preparation(s), if prescribed.
- Moisturiser or foot powder, if required.
- Clean hosiery.

Action	Rationale
Explain each step of any procedure or examination to the patient and gain their consent	Ensures the patient understands the process and encourages their cooperation
Using appropriate moving and handling techniques, assist the patient into a comfortable position – ideally, sitting in a chair at a height where the patient can place their feet on the floor. Alternatively, the patient should lie supine with a pillow under their knees to raise and support the legs	Prevents muscle fatigue and allows the patient to cope with the procedure
Decontaminate hands and put on PPE; gloves can be used if there is a risk of infection or if the patient's skin is broken	Wearing an apron reduces the risk of cross-infection from the nurse's uniform
Ask the patient if they have any feelings of pain, tingling or numbness in the feet or toes	Identifies the possible presence of circulatory problems or neuropathy. If the patient has altered feeling in their feet, they may not notice if the water is too hot or too cold
Fill the basin with warm water and check for temperature using a bath thermometer. Place the basin on top of the disposable pad either on the floor or on the bed within reach of the patient's feet	Reduces the risk of slipping accidents from water on the floor. Reduces the risk of spills onto the bed and having to change linen
Place one of the patient's feet in the basin (check with the patient for water comfort) and wash gently using soap and a washcloth	

Continued

Action	Rationale
Check that the basin is not causing pressure on the patient's legs; if it is, cover the rim with another disposable pad	
Using a washcloth, gently rub any calluses or corns	Removes debris and dead skin. Corns and calluses can cause pain when pressure is applied so any rubbing must be gentle
Wash thoroughly but gently between the toes	Rubbing too hard can cause the skin between the toes to crack and increases the risk of infection
Ask the patient if they would like to soak their feet for a while (unless the patient has diabetes or peripheral vascular disease)	This may feel relaxing to the patient and toenails are softened prior to cutting
Using a jug of warm water (checked for temperature), rinse the foot completely, ensuring that all traces of soap are removed	Soap can be an irritant if left on the skin
Place the patient's foot on a towel and pat dry, paying particular attention to the area between the toes	Failing to dry between the toes causes a breeding ground for bacteria and increases the risk of localised fungal infections, such as athlete's foot
Cover the patient's newly dried foot or put on slipper	The patient's feet may become cold easily, particularly if the patient is older or has circulatory problems
After checking with the patient that the water is still at a comfortable temperature (change the water if necessary), repeat the procedure with the other foot	
Apply (or ask a registered nurse) any prescribed topical care according to prescription to both feet	Skin softener between the toes can cause bacterial infection
OR	
Apply skin softener (avoid using skin softener between the toes)	Massaging skin softener into the feet improves circulation; prevents drying of the skin and makes the skin more flexible (and less prone to cracking)

Action	Rationale
AND/OR	
Apply a **light** dusting of talcum power according to the patient's preferences	Talcum power applied lightly can absorb overproduction of sweat and can ease the process of putting on footwear
Do not at this stage allow the patient to stand	The patient is at greater risk of slipping having had lotion or talcum powder applied to their feet
Assist the patient to put on well-fitting footwear. Ensure socks/tights are not too tight or constrict the circulation. Advise the patient against wearing knee-high tights socks. Shoes/slippers should be well-fitting and secured to the foot without constricting circulation	Restricting circulation to the feet can cause swelling, pain and even blood clots (deep venous thrombosis)
Ask the patient if they have any discomfort and whether can move their toes easily	Being able to move the toes ensures that there is little risk of pressure sores/callus or corn formation from footwear and that circulation will not be affected. Being able to move the toes well also improves balance and reduces the risk of falling
Ensure that the patient is safe and comfortable and has no other requirements	
Clear away all used equipment and dispose of according to local policy; wash and dry the basin thoroughly	
Remove PPE and decontaminate hands	
Document care in the patient's care plan and identify any further evaluation/reassessment/interventions required	Individualises patient care

We tend to take our feet for granted and only pay attention to them when they begin to cause problems. In nursing practice if we fail to care for our patient's feet we risk causing them problems with mobility, infection and pain. Poor care may even lead to the need for amputation. Therefore, nurses must work with the patient to plan the best foot care possible for their needs and recognise the input of other healthcare professionals in maintaining foot health. Nursing interventions should be planned with the goal of informing and assisting the patient towards independence in foot care where possible. However, there are certain groups of patients who should be referred to specialist services, for example podiatry for maintenance of foot and nail health (Box 5.3).

ANATOMY OF THE NAIL

The importance of the fingernail may not be recognised. It is a horny protective structure made of the protein keratin and serves two purposes. The fingernail acts as a protective plate and enhances sensation of the fingertip. The protection function of the fingernail is commonly known but it also has the purpose of enhancing fingertip sensation. The fingertip has many nerve endings and the nail acts in opposition to the fingertip, providing increased sensory input when an object is touched (Mallik, 2004).

The complex nail structure is divided into five specific parts (Fleckman, 2005) (Figure 5.1): the **nail plate**, **nail matrix** (root), **nail bed**, **cuticle** (eponychium) and **nail folds**. Each of these structures has a specific function in nail growth and any problems can result in an abnormal appearance.

Each nail is curved (i.e. convex on its outer surface, concave within). The nail is anchored through the root of the nail being implanted into a groove in the skin. Therefore, part of the nail is under the skin by several millimetres. This portion of the nail does not produce melanin. It is known as the **lunula** (or half moon).

Nail plate

The nail plate is what is thought of as the actual fingernail and is translucent. Blood vessels underneath the nail give it its pink colour. The underneath surface of the nail plate has grooves along the length of the nail that help anchor it to the nail bed. The nail plate is porous to water and the water content is directly related

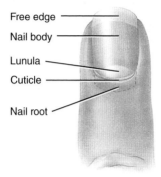

Free edge
Nail body
Lunula
Cuticle
Nail root

Figure 5.1 Dorsal view of a nail. From Tortora GJ, Grabowski SR (2004) *Introduction to the Human Body: Essentials of Anatomy & Physiology*, 6th edn. Reproduced with permission from Wiley-Blackwell.

to it brittleness or hardness. The calcium content of the nail plate is less than 0.5%.

Nail matrix

This is the part of the nail beneath the body and root from which the nail is produced. The matrix (or root) produces keratin cells which make up the nail plate and decide the thickness of the nail. A short matrix produces fewer cells, and as a result a thinner nail; a flat matrix means a flatter nail. The matrix is the most important feature of the nail unit. Damage to the matrix can cause permanent damage to the appearance of the nail.

Nail bed

The nail bed is part of the nail matrix and contains the blood vessels, nerves and melanocytes (or melanin-producing cells). As the nail is produced by the root, it streams down along the nail bed, which adds material to the undersurface of the nail, making it thicker. It is important for normal nail growth that the nail bed is smooth. If it is not, the nail may split or develop grooves.

Cuticle

The cuticle of the fingernail is also called the eponychium. The cuticle fuses the skin of the finger to the nail plate to provide a waterproof barrier and therefore protection for the nail and the underlying skin.

Nail folds

These structures act as a barrier to protect the matrix from damage. The proximal and lateral nail folds are part of the skin that folds at the edges of the nail and continues beneath. Nail folds protect and seal the matrix against bacteria and dirt that could cause infection and damage to the nail bed and plate. Toenails and fingernails have a similar anatomy; however, toenails grow more slowly than fingernails. The rate of nail growth changes throughout life, and the fastest rate occurs during the second decade. Nails tend to grow more quickly in the summer and in warmer climates. Certain illnesses of the immune system can slow nail growth, as can extreme dieting. Medications such as oral steroids and cytotoxins (used as part of chemotherapy) may reduce growth rates. The nails may grow faster in pregnancy, and as a side effect of certain diseases (e.g. psoriasis) or after trauma (Fleckman *et al.*, 2005).

COMMON NAIL DISORDERS

In-growing toenails

This is a common problem resulting for various reasons (e.g. improperly trimmed nails and/or ill-fitting footwear). This condition is most common with the large toenails when part of the nail plate pierces the lateral nail fold. The exaggerated curvature may gradually grow into the lateral nail fold and produce pain (Alavi *et al.*, 2007). Often the first sign is pain, but infection is a high risk, as is eventual difficulty with walking. Proper shoes with an ample toe box (front of the shoe) should be worn to remove pressure from the lateral nail folds. The patient should be instructed to cut the nails straight across and not to cut them too short.

Table 5.2 Nail discoloration

Discoloration	Associated condition
Green finger/toenails	Infection: usually pseudomonas
Brown fingernails	Often a sign of exposure to chemicals through occupations. Nicotine may also stain the nail and surrounding finger a yellowish-brown colour
Yellow finger/toenails	Thyroid problems or lymphoedema
Red/black finger/toenails	Often caused by trauma and bruising of the nail bed (subungal haemorrhage) In severe cases the nail will detach from the nail bed
Black finger/toenails	Symptomatic of vitamin B12 deficiency
Opaque white (distal half)/ pinkish-brown (proximal half) finger/toenails	Symptomatic of chronic renal failure
Opaque white finger/toenails	Signifies chronic disease, e.g. cardiac failure, cirrhosis of the liver or diabetes in people aged over 50 years

(*Source:* Scher *et al.*, 2003)

Clinically, the most common nail disorders can be classified into five groups based on the most salient presenting features (Alavi *et al.*, 2007):

- Nail discoloration (Table 5.2).
- Nail thickening: caused by trauma, poor circulation or normal ageing.
- Nail surface abnormalities (Box 5.4).
- Inflammation of the nail fold.
- Nail fungal infection.

Inflammation of the nail fold (paronychia)

This is characterised by inflammation of the tissue around the fingernail. Pus accumulates between the cuticle and the nail matrix and is often caused by bacterial infection. People with psoriasis or eczema often have a chronic form of paronychia. Topical steroids have been found to be more effective than oral medication for the treatment of the condition (Tosti *et al.*, 2002).

Box 5.4 Nail surface abnormalities

- Longitudinal ridging: may be due to rheumatoid arthritis or peripheral vascular disease (circulatory problems). Can also be associated with alopecia and is a normal sign of ageing.
- Transverse ridging: usually due to a temporary disturbance of nail growth, e.g. acute illness. The condition is usually not long term.
- Finger clubbing: an increase in the soft tissue of the distal part of the fingers or toes. Is associated with chronic lung disease, e.g. emphysema or cystic fibrosis.
- Pitting: nail pitting is associated with psoriasis, which will affect the nail in about 50% of people with the condition. Alopecia can also present with nail pitting.

(*Source:* Scher *et al.*, 2003)

Fungal nail infections
Onychomycosis (fungal infection of the toenail(s)

Fungal nail infections occur when fungi and yeast colonise the nails and nail beds. Onychomycosis is a chronic disorder affecting the structure of the nail (Baran *et al.*, 1999). Although the finger-nails can be affected, there is a much higher incidence involving toenails (Alavi *et al.*, 2007). This is one of the most prevalent skin conditions and is primarily found in older people, although conditions such as psoriasis and any illnesses which lower the immune system increase the risk of developing fungal infections of the nails – usually the toenails. People with diabetes are particularly vulnerable to fungal infection and, compared to the general population, the responsible organism is likely to be different.

There are three main clinical forms of onychomycosis (Box 5.5) which present with the following symptoms (Eliopoulos, 2001):

- Cracks and/or fissures between the toes.
- Thickened and hardened toenails.
- Abnormally shaped toenails.
- Toenails may become detached from the nail bed.
- Toenails become brittle and flaky.

> **Box 5.5 The three main types of onychomycosis**
>
> - Distolateral subungual onychomycosis: the commonest form where fungus advances from an infection of the adjacent skin into the nail bed, the nail plate and, in advanced cases, the nail matrix. This form can also be subject to secondary bacterial infection.
> - White superficial onychomycosis: caused by the dermatophyte *Trichophyton mentagrophytes*. The nail surface is infected, whereas the rest of the nail plate, the nail bed and the matrix remain unaltered.
> - Proximal subungual onychomycosis: this less common form starts with an infection of the skin of the proximal nail fold (at the base of the nail) and spreads to the nail plate and the matrix.
>
> (*Source:* Bell-Syer *et al.*, 2002)

The condition can cause psychological distress due to its unattractive appearance. Physically, the patient can be affected by pain or toenail discomfort, which can affect mobility. Injury to the surrounding skin may allow bacterial infection, resulting in cellulitis, osteomyelitis, sepsis and tissue necrosis. Such complications seem to occur more frequently in older people and in people with diabetes mellitus (Blumberg & Cantor, 2005). Only 20–50% of suspected nail infections are found to be caused by parasitic fungi attacking the skin; there are other causes, such as direct trauma to the nail (wearing shoes that are too tight, nail biting), poor peripheral circulation, psoriasis, lichen planus, diabetes or poor foot care (Faergemann & Baran, 2003).

All the above conditions will require referral to a podiatrist. Nurses should not take the initiative to carry out toenail care without specialist advice and intervention.

NURSING MANAGEMENT

Some people will be prescribed oral medication for several months to eradicate the infection (British National Formulary, 2009). Toenail infections will take longer to clear up than fingernail infections will. People with less severe infections, which only affect the distal part of the nail, can be treated with topical preparations or nail paints. General advice that nurses should offer to patients includes:

- Wash and thoroughly dry feet every day – do not over soak (skin becomes soggy and prone to injury/infection).
- Avoid tight-fitting shoes (friction may cause skin breaks, which can become infected).
- Wear leather shoes (allows the feet to breathe and cuts down sweat).
- Wear cotton socks that are not tight (cotton allows the feet to breathe and tight socks can add pressure to the nails, which can cause symptoms similar to fungal infection).
- Change socks every day (keeps the feet clean and eradicates the infection).
- Trim nails regularly (nails cut frequently are less prone to prolonged infection times).

CUTTING FINGER- AND TOENAILS

Nails should be clean, short and smooth. Fingernails with dirt underneath spread infection and ragged fingernails can cause injury and infection. Nail care is done best when the person is sitting in a chair. If the person is not able to sit in a chair, it can be done in the bed. Nurses are expected to undertake toenail care, which previously may have been done by chiropody services. However, there are exceptions to nurses cutting nails where the procedure is unsafe and may put the patient at risk. If there is any doubt about safety, refer to the registered nurse or specialist health professional. In the following circumstances, the podiatrist should undertake the care and nursing staff should not attempt any nail cutting/trimming procedures.

- Any nails which are thickened, horned, misshapen or have evidence of disease.
- Patients who have type 1 or type 2 diabetes.
- Patients who have any circulatory problems.
- Patients who have any neurological conditions that affect the sensation in their feet.
- Patients who are on anticoagulant therapy (blood-thinning medication).
- Patients who are immunosuppressed, e.g. chemotherapy, HIV.

- Any patient who has a cognitive deficit and who cannot understand to cooperate with the procedure.
- Patients who wear any orthotic support.
- Any patients who have a foot trauma.
- Patients who have foot deformities that impede access to the toenails.

Procedure: Cutting toenails
Equipment

- Bowl with warm water and bath thermometer.
- Liquid soap or oil.
- Disposable scissors.
- Disposable (or sterilised) long-handled nail nippers.
- Orange stick or cotton buds.
- Towel.
- Nail file.
- Hand cream.
- Disposable waste bag.

Action	Rationale
Explain each step of any procedure or examination to the patient and gain their consent	Ensures the patient understands the process and encourages their cooperation
If the patient is not freshly out of a bath/shower, the toenails will need to be soaked	
Gather equipment and place it on a trolley or flat surface	
Decontaminate hands	
Fill a bowl with warm water (up to 43°C) and add a small amount of liquid soap or oil	Loosens any dirt under the fingernails
Soak the feet for a short time – no more than 10 minutes	Longer than 10 minutes makes the feet soft and more prone to injury
Dry the feet, toes and between the toes	Wet feet and nails may cause the nurse to slip from the finger being attended to and cause injury. Wet nails may be ragged when cut

Continued

Action	Rationale
Sweep a swab soaked in 0.5% chlorhexidine solution over the toenails	Cleans the skin and will prevent bacterial invasion if the foot is accidentally injured
Sit at a level equal to the patient or elevate the bed to a comfortable working height	
Place a sheet of paper under the patient's foot to collect the cut toenails	
If right-handed, hold the toe between the fingers of your left hand and pull the fleshy part of the toe slightly away from the nail	Prevents accidental nipping of the skin round the nail
Starting at the outside of the nail make small nips in the nail across to the other side, following the shape of the nail	
Do not cut down the side of the nail	Encourages in-grown toenails
Do not cut too short	
Use a nail file to shape the nails into a square shape – but do not leave sharp edges. **NB:** if toenails are too thick to cut, file down into shape	Sharp edges will dig into the toes when shoes are worn
File in one direction – from the outer edge of the nail towards the middle	Filing back and forth weakens the nail and can also make the nail jagged
The finished nail should feel smooth to the touch	Jagged nails can accidentally scratch the skin or catch on clothes, which can cause nails to tear or break
Repeat for all nails	
Check the nails for signs of abnormalities and ask the patient if they have any concerns	
Swab the toenails with 0.5% chlorhexidine or alcohol gel	Prevents the spread of infection
Apply any topical preparations and/or massage cream into the foot (avoiding between the toes)	
Clear away and dispose of used equipment according to local policy	
Return the patient to a comfortable position and ensure they have access to the nurse call system	
Decontaminate hands	
Document the care, noting any areas of concern and for further assessment	

Procedure: Cutting fingernails

Equipment

- Bowl with warm water and bath thermometer.
- Liquid soap or oil.
- Disposable (or sterilised) long-handled nail nippers.
- 0.5% chlorhexidine solution.
- Towel.
- Paper sheet to collect debris.
- Sterile swabs.
- Sterile nail file.
- Disposable waste bag.

Action	Rationale
Explain each step of any procedure or examination to the patient and gain their consent	Ensures the patient understands the process and encourages their cooperation
If the patient is not freshly out of a bath/ shower, the fingernails will need to be soaked	
Gather equipment and place it on a trolley or flat surface	
Decontaminate hands	
Fill a bowl with warm water (up to 43°C) and add a small amount of liquid soap or oil	Loosens any dirt under the fingernails
Soak the fingertips for a short time – no more than five minutes	Longer than five minutes makes the finger tips soft and more prone to injury
Dry the hands and nails	Wet hands and nails may cause the nurse to slip from the finger being attended to and cause injury. Wet nails may be ragged when cut
Sit at a level equal to the patient or elevate the bed to a comfortable working height	
Gently use an orange stick or preferably a cotton bud to remove dirt from under the nails	These implements are softer than a nail brush and carry less risk of injury or infection

Continued

Action	Rationale
Cut or nip nails straight across the finger tip to the end of the finger or just beyond, depending on patient preference	Cutting too short risks cutting the skin
Use a nail file to shape the nails into an oval shape – not pointed	Pointed nails break easily. Filing too low down the side of the nails weakens the nail
File in one direction – from the outer edge of the nail towards the middle on both sides of the nail in long sweeps. **NB:** do not file in a seesaw motion	Filing back and forth weakens the nail and can make the nail jagged
The finished nail should follow the contour of the quick and feel smooth to the touch	Jagged nails can accidentally scratch the skin or catch on clothes, which can cause nails to tear or break
Repeat for all nails	
Check the nails for signs of abnormalities and ask the patient if they have any concerns	
Massage hand cream into the hands and nails	Nourishes the fingernails and promotes comfort for the patient
Check the feet for any conditions which require referral to specialist staff	
Clear away and dispose of used equipment according to local policy	
Return the patient to a comfortable position and ensure they have access to the nurse call system	
Decontaminate hands	
Document the care, noting any areas of concern and for further assessment	

CONCLUSION

Although people in general take great care of their bodies and their faces, for example shaving, applying make-up and moisturisers etc., many people ignore their feet until their feet become problematic. This chapter demonstrates the importance of assessing patient's feet for disease processes or abnormalities. This is vital if patients are to be able to mobilise and remain pain-free while doing so. Nursing staff should be aware of the advice they can give for maintaining healthy feet and finger- and toenails and incorporate foot and nail care into the fundamental care activities they carry out with the patient.

REFERENCES

Alavi A, Woo K, Sibbald RG (2007) Common nail disorders and fungal infections. *Advances in Skin and Wound Care* **20**(6): 346–357.

American Diabetes Association (2008) Diagnosis and classification of diabetes mellitus. *Diabetes Care* **31**(suppl. 1): S55–S60.

American Podiatric Medical Association (2009) About podiatry, http://www.apma.org/MainMenu/Foot-Health/FootHealthBrochures/GeneralFootHealthBrochures.aspx, [accessed 10 April 2009].

Badlissi F, Dunn JE, Link CL *et al.* (2005) Foot musculoskeletal disorders, pain, and foot-related functional limitation in older persons. *Journal of the American Geriatrics Society* **53**(6): 1029–1033.

Baker N, Murali-Krishnan S, Fowler D (2005a) A user's guide to foot screening: Part 2: Peripheral arterial disease. *The Diabetic Foot* **8**(2), http://findarticles.com/p/articles/mi_m0MDQ/is_2_8/ai_n15396892 [accessed 3 April 2009].

Baker N, Murali-Krishnan S, Rayman G (2005b) A user's guide to foot screening: Part 1: Peripheral neuropathy. *The Diabetic Foot* **8**(1), http://findarticles.com/p/articles/mi_m0MDQ/is_1_8/ai_n13496122/, [accessed 3 April 2009].

Baran R, Hay R, Haneke E *et al.* (1999) *Onychomycosis: The current approach to diagnosis and treatment*. Martin Dunitz, London.

Bell-Syer SEM, Hart R, Crawford F *et al.* (2002) Oral treatments for fungal infections of the skin of the foot. *Cochrane Database of Systematic Reviews* Issue 2, Art. No.: CD003584. DOI: 10.1002/14651858. CD003584

Blumberg M, Cantor G (2005) Onychomycosis, http://emedicine.medscape.com/article/1105828-overview, [accessed 8 March 2009].

British National Formulary (2009) *British National Formulary*, 58th edn. Pharmaceuticals Press, London.

Brookes S, O'Leary B (2006) Feet first: A guide to diabetic foot services. *British Journal of Nursing* **15**(15): S4–S10.

Bryant J, Beinlich N (1999) Foot care: Focus on the elderly. *Orthopaedic Nursing* **18**(6): 53–60.

Burrow JG (2004) An overview of foot care for older people. *Nursing & Residential Care* **6**(3): 120–123.

Chamley CA, Carson P, Randall D *et al.* (2005) *Developmental anatomy and physiology of children*. Elsevier, London.

Crawford F, Hollis S (2008) Topical treatments for fungal infections of the skin and nails of the foot. *Cochrane Database of Systematic Reviews 2008 Issue 4*. John Wiley & Sons, Chichester.

Department of Health (1994) *Feet First: Report of the Joint Department of Health and NHS Chiropody Task Force*. NHS Executive, Leeds.

Department of Health (2001) *The Essence of Care: Patient-focused benchmarking for health care practitioners*. DH, London.

Department of Health (2008) *Podiatry: Care services efficiency delivery*. DH, London.

Diabetes UK (2008) Long term complications, http://www.diabetes.org.uk/Guide-to-diabetes/Complications/Long_term_complications/, [accessed 22 October 2009].

Diabetes UK (2004) *Diabetes in the UK*. Diabetes UK, London.

Dickson N, Wright P, Woodrow P (2008) *Toe-nail and Foot Care for Non-diabetic Adults: Guidelines for nursing staff and Allied Health Professionals*. East Kent NHS Trust.

Edmonds ME, Foster AVM (2006) Diabetic foot ulcers. *British Medical Journal* **332**(7538): 407–410.

Edwards M (2008) Risk reduction and care for the diabetic foot. *Practice Nurse* **36**(4): **21**, 23–24, 26.

Eliopoulos C (2001) *Gerontological Nursing*, 5th edn. Lippincott, Philadelphia.

Faergemann J, Baran R (2003) Epidemiology, clinical presentation and diagnosis of onychomycosis. *British Journal of Dermatology* **149** (suppl. 65): 1–4.

Fleckman P (2005) Structure and function of the nail unit. In: RK Scher, CR Daniel III (eds), *Nails: Diagnosis, therapy, surgery*. Elsevier Saunders, Oxford, 14–25.

Fletcher J (2006) Full nursing assessment of patients at risk of diabetic foot ulcers. *British Journal of Nursing* (suppl. 'Tissue Viability') **15**(15): S18–S21.

Frey C (2000) Foot health and shoewear for women. *Clinical Orthopaedics and Related Research* **372**: 32–44.

George M (1995) Chiropody services: A feat for nursing? *Nursing Standard* **9**(31): 22.

Kravitz SR, McGuire J, Shanahan SD (2003) Physical assessment of the diabetic foot. *Advances in Skin & Wound Care* **16**(2): 68–75.

Leese G, Schofield C, McMurray B *et al.* (2007) Scottish foot ulcer risk score predicts foot ulcer healing in a regional specialist foot clinic. *Diabetes Care* **30**(8): 2064–2069.

Mallik M (2004) Hygiene. In: M Mallik, C Hall, D Howard (eds), *Nursing Knowledge and Practice*, Elsevier, London, 281–303.

Mayfield JA, Reiber GE, Sanders LJ (1998) Preventive foot care in people with diabetes (Technical Review). *Diabetes Care* **21**(12): 2161–2177.

Menz HB, Lord SR (2001a) Foot pain impairs balance and functional ability in community-dwelling older people. *Journal of the American Podiatric Medical Association* **91**(5): 262–268.

Menz HB, Lord SR (2001b) The contribution of foot problems to mobility impairment and falls in community-dwelling older people. *Journal of the American Geriatrics Society* **49**(12): 1651–1656.

National Institute for Health and Clinical Excellence (2008) *Type 2 Diabetes: The management of type 2 diabetes (NICE guideline)*. NICE, London.

Scher R, Fleckman P, Tulumbus B *et al.* (2003) Brittle nail syndrome: Treatment options and the role of the nurse. *Dermatology Nursing* **15**(1): 15–23.

Sheehan P, Jones P, Caselli A (2003) Percent change in wound area of diabetic foot ulcers over a 4-week period is a robust predictor of complete healing in a 12-week prospective trial. *Diabetes Care* **26**(6): 1879–1882.

Thomson P, Volpe RG, Wernick J (2001) *Introduction to Podopaediatrics*, 2nd edn. Churchill Livingstone, London.

Tosti A, Piraccini BM, Ghetti E *et al.* (2002) Topical steroids versus systemic antifungals in the treatment of chronic paronychia: An open, randomized double-blind and double-dummy study. *Journal of the American Academy of Dermatology* **47**(1): 73–76.

Williams AE, Nester CJ, Ravey MI (2008) Rheumatoid arthritis patients' experiences of wearing therapeutic footwear: A qualitative investigation. *BMC Musculoskeletal Disorders* **8**: 104, http://www.biomedcentral.com/1471-2474/8/104, [accessed 20 October 2009].

Hair Care and Grooming | **6**

THE IMPORTANCE OF HAIR CARE

Hair has three main purposes: retaining body temperature to ensure survival, transmitting important sensory information to the brain and expressing gender identity. Throughout history, hair has symbolised attractiveness and sex appeal (Batchelor, 2001) as well as highlighting religious and cultural beliefs (Williams, 1995). Hair on the body is associated with growth and maturity and its natural variations are important to self-image (Sinclair, 2007). Shiny hair with a smooth texture is generally perceived to be healthy and attractive. Hair texture and shine relate to hair surface properties, whereas the integrity and health of hair ends relates to the hair cortex. Hair varies in type and colour. Cosmetics are used widely to alter the properties of hair, for example artificial colouring or alteration of the normal structure (e.g. straightening) as dictated by culture and fashion (Sinclair, 2007).

The aim of this chapter is to help the reader understand how to carry out hair care and the underpinning rationale(s) for care.

LEARNING OUTCOMES

After reading this chapter, the reader will be able to:

❑ Describe the anatomy and physiology of hair.
❑ Identify common diseases of the scalp and hair during assessment.
❑ Assess for factors impacting on maintaining a healthy scalp.
❑ Understand and carry out clinical care of the patient's hair.
❑ Assess for factors impacting on hair removal.

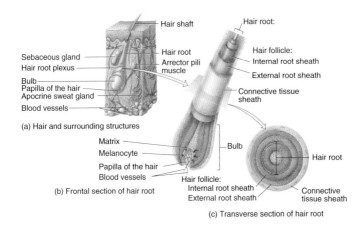

Hair shaft

Hair root:

Sebaceous gland
Hair root plexus

Hair root
Arrector pili
muscle

Hair follicle:
Internal root sheath
External root sheath

Bulb
Papilla of the hair
Apocrine sweat gland
Blood vessels

Connective tissue
sheath

(a) Hair and surrounding structures

Matrix
Melanocyte
Papilla of the hair
Blood vessels

Bulb

Hair root

(b) Frontal section of hair root

Hair follicle:
Internal root sheath
External root sheath

Connective
tissue sheath

(c) Transverse section of hair root

Figure 6.1 Anatomy of the hair. From Tortora GJ, Grabowski SR (2004) *Introduction to the Human Body; Essentials of Anatomy & Physiology*, 6th edn. Reproduced with permission from Wiley-Blackwell.

❏ Understand the evidence base underpinning clinical procedures.

ANATOMY OF THE HAIR

Hair has two separate structures: the **follicle** and the **shaft** (Figure 6.1). The follicle is a layered structure with many functions. The base of the follicle – the **dermal papilla** – is a projection filled with blood vessels; surrounding the papilla is the only living part of the hair: the **bulb**. **Sensory nerve fibres** surrounding the bulb alert a person when the hair is moved. Each follicle has **sebaceous glands** that secrete oil to condition the hair and the surrounding skin. Hair colour is determined by **pigmented cells** (melanocytes), growing at the dermal papilla.

The follicle is surrounded by two hair sheaths, which protect the growing hair follicle. The **inner sheath** ends below the **sweat gland** and the **outer sheath** extends further up to the **apocrine** (scent) **glands**. The **arrector pili** muscle attaches the gland to the fibrous layer of the sheath, which can cause the hair to stand up when stimulated (e.g. when in a cold environment or when frightened). The muscle contracting causes the hair to be pulled downwards so it stands up straight (goose bumps).

The triple layered shaft of the hair comprises keratin. The inner and middle layers – the **medulla** and **cortex** – dictate hair thickness. The outer layer – the **cuticle** – comprises several overlapping scales which when in good condition improve the appearance of the hair.

The cross-sectional shape of the hair determines wave and curl, how much light hair can deflect (shine) and the amount of sebum retained. This determines the appearance of the hair and its perceived manageability (Draelos, 2005).

Hair is porous and absorbs water. When wet, hair can be stretched by up to 30% without damage, but hair will break if stretched beyond 80% (Dawber & Messenger, 1997). Although hair grows at an average rate of 2 mm per week, it undergoes different phases of growth. Actively growing hair is anagen; resting hair is labelled telogen hair; after resting, it naturally sheds (falls out).

THE INFLUENCE OF LIFESPAN ON HAIR HEALTH AND HYGIENE

Infancy (0–23 months)

Downy hair appears during the months of gestation (before birth) and is gradually replaced in the first few months of life (Chamley *et al.*, 2005). Poor nutrition at any age will influence the rate and amount of hair growth. Babies should have their hair/head shampooed daily using small amounts of very mild shampoo. This will prevent the onset of seborrhoea (cradle cap).

Childhood (2–12 years)

All downy hair is gradually replaced, while genetics decide the colour, thickness, coarseness and distribution of hair. The risk of infestation by head lice is high, including re-infestation after treatment. Head lice affect approximately 2% of school-age children at any one time. During the treatment phase, activities such as swimming within 48 hours after treatment reduce the effectiveness of some treatments to eradicate head lice (Health Protection Agency, 2005).

For children with childhood cancers, the loss of hair as a side effect of treatment(s) can cause psychological problems and their feelings should be taken into account during treatment.

Adolescence (13–19 years)

With the onset of puberty, hormonal changes result in growth spurts and the appearance of body hair. In the early stages of puberty, pubic hair will develop as a soft downy pale layer over the base of the scrotum and phallus in boys and labia majora (outer lips) of the vagina in girls. As puberty progresses, the pubic hair will become denser and more pigmented until, at the final stage of puberty, it will resemble that of adults (Neinstein & Kaufman, 2002). Excessive hair growth in adolescents has different causes (Table 6.1) but distresses teenagers, who are already having to become accustomed to other body changes associated with puberty.

Teenagers may complain of hair loss when there appears to be no particular cause or disease process. This may be due to telogen effluvium (hair loss of the telogen phase), where the teenager has

Table 6.1 Abnormal hair growth and patterns beginning in adolescence

Type of abnormal hair growth	Pattern of hair growth	Cause(s)
Hirsutism: excessive growth of coarse hair not normal female pattern growth	Hair grows over upper abdomen, chest and face	Ovulatory disorders
Hypertrichosis: excessive growth of normal hair	Normal pattern	Side effect of anticonvulsant medication
Virilisation	Presents as hirsutism but with androgen excess (excessive growth of hair)	May be associated with rare malignancy

had an illness previously (e.g. glandular fever or even pregnancy) when the hair has gone into the resting phase. As the teenager recovers, the hair begins to grow normally again, causing shedding of telogen hairs at around 3–5 times the usual rate. This usually resolves in 3–6 months (Neinstein, 2004).

Adolescent boys may start to worry after noticing some receding near the temples. This normal development does not mean they are losing hair; their hairlines are merely developing from the straight-across boys' pattern to the more M-shaped pattern of adult men.

Adulthood (20–64 years)

Females may lose their hair after childbirth due to the same telogen effluvium found in teenagers. However, throughout adulthood, everybody loses hair to some extent but usually it is more apparent in men. Common baldness is known as androgenic alopecia, which implies that a combination of hormones and heredity (genetics) underpins the condition. In male pattern baldness, there is rarely the rapid shedding of hair in telogen effluvium but hair is not replaced.

Women also have a genetic tendency to lose hair, but the female pattern is more diffuse, with less likelihood of the frontal hairline being lost. Male pattern baldness in women implies a hormone imbalance. The menstrual cycle has also been found to affect perceptions of hair growth (Birch & Messenger, 2003).

Older age (65+ years)

Ageing results in a reduced production of melanin by the hair follicles, hence the hair begins to grey (although this is not restricted to older people). Like skin changes, hair becomes drier and more brittle with ageing. The texture of hair also changes and greyer hair tends to be coarse.

Female facial hair is likely to increase, usually because the finer and lighter hair covering the face is replaced by more prominent and darker hair. Women may choose to remove this facial hair using depilatory creams rather than shaving as shaving stimulates hair growth and the hair is rougher to the touch.

THE EFFECT OF DEPENDENCE IN ACHIEVING HAIR HEALTH AND HYGIENE

Patients who are unconscious or those with mobility and dexterity problems will be unable to care for their hair independently. The act of brushing and shampooing the hair stimulates circulation to the scalp and removes dirt. If the patient is unable to undertake self-care, their hair may become dirty and/or matted.

PHYSICAL FACTORS INFLUENCING HAIR HEALTH

The hair is a fairly accurate measure of general health status. Hair cells are some of the fastest growing in the body, and when the body is under stress or in crisis (e.g. owing to acute illness, pregnancy or the menopause) hair cells can shut down in order to redirect energy elsewhere. Physical conditions causing hair loss include hormonal changes, nutritional deficiencies, a variety of medications, surgery and medical conditions, in particular, thyroid disease. Hair loss may also be associated with fungal infection or autoimmune alopecia (see below), involving circular patches of hair loss that require referral to a dermatologist.

Generally, hair and scalp disorders are not associated with any systemic biological impairment. However, given hair's important role in determining self-image, social perception and psychosocial functioning, hair and scalp disorders can prove distressing for both men and women.

PSYCHOLOGICAL FACTORS INFLUENCING HAIR HEALTH

Hair appearance is crucial to self-esteem, particularly for women. Most people underestimate the psychological effects of hair loss in women, who may feel that their condition is not taken seriously (Birch *et al.*, 2006). Hair is an important reflection of self-image for both sexes and a significant number of men report fear of losing their hair. Men with increased hair loss demonstrate greater dissatisfaction with their appearance (Girman *et al.*, 1998). However, balding is a more typical, and less noticeable, part of the appearance in older age (Rexbye *et al.*, 2005).

SOCIOCULTURAL FACTORS INFLUENCING HAIR HEALTH AND HYGIENE

Hair structure varies between cultures (McMichael, 2007). Black African hair is easily traumatised and broken. Careful handling using specialist shampoos and conditioners such as wheat germ oil or lanolin is recommended (Dawber, 1996). Conditioner increases manageability, decreases grooming friction and adds shine.

The processes of dressing hair can affect its health; tight braiding of hair can cause traction alopecia at the temples (Sinclair *et al.*, 1999). Although straightening hair can make it easier to manage, the side effects of straightening can cause scarring alopecia (Draelos, 1997) ,which results in permanent hair loss, also known as hot comb alopecia procedures (Sinclair *et al.*, 1999).

Asian hair is more resistant than Caucasian to environmental damage because of its thicker cuticle layer (Beom *et al.*, 2006).

Hair removal by both sexes dates back to the days of cavemen (Mehmi & Abdullah, 2007). Females in this country are expected to remove hair from their legs, underarms and, more recently, pubic region, whereas European women and men find the natural unshaved look acceptable.

Throughout the Islamic world, hair removal is set within the context of religious law. Muslim men and women may wish to remove their armpit and pubic hair. However, men are expected to keep their facial hair, although females can remove unwanted facial hair but should not change the shape of their eyebrows. The Sikh religion forbids any hair cutting as the growing and maintenance of long hair reflects the strength of their religious beliefs. Judaism prohibits the use of razor blades, but electric shavers may be used. Other religions encourage the shaving of the head (e.g. Buddhism).

ENVIRONMENTAL FACTORS INFLUENCING HAIR HEALTH

The fashion for hair extensions strains hair health. Glue from the extensions prevents normal shedding of telogen hairs, which then attach to the extension, resulting in acute hair matting. The risk of traction alopecia is thought to be significant but under-reported.

The presence of alopecia associated with the siting of the extensions has been found 7-20 days after having extensions (Yang *et al.*, 2009).

Sunburn, air pollution and chlorine-contaminated water all stress the hair.

POLITICO-ECONOMIC FACTORS INFLUENCING HAIR HEALTH

There are few factors relating to this category that would directly affect hair health. The main political factors relates to equality and the right in certain religions and faiths to cover the head. Nurses must be aware of those faiths whose strictures prevent the exposure of the body without a chaperone or to carers of a specific gender.

GENERAL ASSESSMENT OF HAIR HEALTH AND HYGIENE

Diseases of the hair rarely impact on abilities to carry out other activities of living (ALs). However, problems with maintaining body temperature, of poor nutrition and reduced mobility can all affect a person's hair health and/or ability to self-care (Table 6.2).

Safety issues

As with any procedure that involves the use of water, water temperature must be monitored. This may be in a basin, shower or shower attachments in baths. Hair washing can cause water to splash over the sides of basins or over a bathroom floor. Therefore, there is a risk of slips and falls. Where possible, non-slip mats should be provided for patients who are self-caring. Nurses washing patients' hair in bed should take particular care against splashing especially if there is any electrical equipment in the vicinity.

Infection control measures

The same measures are required for hair washing as for any procedure which involves the use of either water receptacles (e.g. basins) or communal washing areas (e.g. showers or bathrooms).

Table 6.2 The assessment of activities of living and hair hygiene

Activity of living	Assessment
Maintaining a safe environment	Can the patient safely manage to care for their hair?
	Does the patient understand how to carry out hair hygiene?
	Is the patient too ill/in too much pain to carry out self-care?
Mobilising	Are any mobility aids required to increase the safety of the patient while carrying out hair hygiene, e.g. a chair, safety bar?
Eating and drinking	Does the patient require any nutritional supplements to improve hair health?
Eliminating	Does the patient have any problems with incontinence and pubic hygiene?
Maintaining body temperature	Does the patient have a temperature, which may cause sweating?
Working and playing	Does the patient have any infestation that requires infection control measures before interacting with others?
	Does the patient feel that their appearance relating to their hair/scalp health and/or hygiene impacts on their self-confidence when interacting with others?
	What measures must be taken to ensure that the patient's spiritual and cultural needs are met?
Expressing sexuality	What are the patient's normal hair care/hair dressing practices?
	What products does the patient prefer?
Dying	Are there any spiritual or religious requirements that must be met as part of 'end of life' care?

Moving and handling

For patients who require assistance in managing hair hygiene, a full manual handling assessment should be carried out to ensure the patient's and nurse's safety.

Prescribed care

Patients may be prescribed topical treatments in the form of shampoos and scalp preparations, for example treating head lice, dermatitis and psoriasis of the scalp.

COMMON HAIR CONDITIONS
Head lice (*Pediculosis capitis*)

Head lice are parasites, tiny greyish-brown, wingless insects that most commonly infest the scalps of school-age children, although adults also get them.

Lice attach their eggs (nits) to hair shafts near the scalp, behind the ears and at the back of the neck. Hatched eggshells may be confused with dandruff. The mature louse is 204 mm long with hook-like claws on six legs that grasp the strand of hair tightly, making it difficult to dislodge. Most people who are infested are unaware as most cases are asymptomatic. Itching and tiny red spots are caused by the louse feeding on the host's blood. Itching may not present for some time after infestation or may persist after treatment due to a hyper-sensitive reaction (allergy) to lice saliva (Sladden & Johnston, 2004). Severe infestation runs to thousands of lice, but typical infestations have about 30 lice per head (Speare & Canyon, 2005).

The diagnosis of lice infestation can be made definitively only if living lice are present (Nash, 2003). The most effective method to detect and dislodge live lice is to run a fine-toothed comb through the hair and wipe onto a light-coloured cover/wrap over the shoulders.

Infestation can be treated using lotions or liquid preparations. Alcohol-based formulations are effective, but water-based formulations are preferred for small children and patients with asthma or eczema.

A contact time of 12 hours or overnight treatment is recommended for lotions and liquids; a two-hour treatment is not sufficient to kill eggs (British National Formulary, 2009). Precautions with clothing and bedding are not needed, as lice cannot survive away from the hair.

It is not recommended that lice treatments be used routinely, as lice become immune. Bug busting or the combing method – wet hair with conditioner – is becoming more popular and effective for school children.

Procedure: Wet combing method for detection of head lice and elimination of lice (bug busting)

Equipment (detection)

- Ordinary comb (patient's or disposable).
- Personal protective equipment (PPE).
- Fine-toothed (nit) comb.
- Disposal bag.
- Plastic draw sheet or paper cover (light-coloured/white).
- Relevant manual handling equipment.

Equipment (elimination)

As above plus:

- Disposable polythene sheet.
- Complete change of bed linen and patient's clothing.
- Clinical waste bag.
- Disposable cap in case of severe infestation.

Action	Rationale
Explain each step of any procedure or examination to the patient and gain their consent	Ensures the patient understands the process and encourages their cooperation
Place patient in most appropriate and comfortable position using manual handling techniques and equipment as determined through assessment	The patient will be able to tolerate the procedure if comfortable
Decontaminate hands and wear appropriate PPE	Prevents cross-infection
Detecting head lice (most effective on freshly washed hair)	
Cover the patient's shoulders or pillow with a light-coloured wrap	Detects the dropping of lice from the hair or comb
Comb hair into sections using an ordinary comb	Increases visual detection of lice
Examine for lice or nits by running a fine-toothed (detector) comb from the root to the end of the hair	

Action	Rationale
Wipe the comb on a light-coloured surface after each sweep and inspect for eggs or live lice	Detects the presence of head lice and the affected area of the scalp
If lice are detected, sensitively inform the patient and refer to medical staff for prescribed care	
Document in patient's notes and refer to a prescriber for topical treatment	
Eliminating head lice	
Avoiding contact with the eyes, apply prescribed preparation according to the pharmacist's/manufacturer's instructions	Preparations are usually toxic. Ensures maximum effectiveness of the preparation
Massage or comb through the hair checking for sensitivity to the preparation	
Allow hair to dry naturally and, if necessary, shampoo after the time identified as required for lotion application and effectiveness	
OR	
Wash hair as normal using water at the correct temperature and apply conditioner liberally	Head lice lose their grip on the hair
Comb the hair through with a normal comb	Reduces tangling and hair breakage
Comb hair into sections	Allows methodical removal of lice/ nits
Run a fine-toothed (detector) comb from the root to the end of the hair	Dislodges the lice from the hair shaft
Wipe the comb on a light-coloured surface after each sweep	Removes the lice and prevents moving them to other areas of the scalp
Work over the whole head for at least 30 minutes	Ensures that all areas of the scalp have been treated
Rinse the hair using normal products	
Return the patient to their preferred position and ensure comfort	
Clear away used equipment into clinical waste	
Decontaminate hands	Prevents cross-infection
Record in patients notes and arrange follow-up treatment if appropriate	Allows evaluation of care

If using conditioner, the procedure should be repeated every three days for at least two weeks. If using a prescribed preparation, the procedure would usually be repeated after seven days. (**NB:** hair should be treated only if a live louse has been detected and **never** as a precaution against head lice.)

Tea tree conditioner has been identified as a useful alternative therapy, but to date there has been no medical evidence to support its use over normal conditioner.

Pubic lice (*Phthirus pubis*)

Pubic infestation is usually through sexual contact (Scott, 2001). Lice live on coarse hair, notably in the pubic and perianal areas, but can also be found on the eyelashes, abdomen, back, in the axillae and on the head if hair is coarse and widely spaced. They cause itching for the same reasons as head lice but are easier to detect because of the itchy red papules, which are often worse at night. Scatterings of tiny dark-brown specks (louse excreta) may also be found on the skin and underwear (Wendel & Rompalo, 2002). Treatment is usually through referral to the GUM (genitourinary medicine) clinic, where an insecticide will be prescribed for eradication. Patients will normally be screened for signs of other sexually transmitted diseases and advised to avoid sexual or close body contact for the duration of the treatment (Royal College of General Practitioners, 2006).

Seborrhoeic dermatitis

Seborrhoeic dermatitis (Figure 6.2) is a chronic inflammatory disorder affecting areas of the head and trunk, where sebaceous glands are most prominent. The distribution is often symmetrical, and common sites of involvement are the hairy areas of the head and face. Other sites include the forehead, between the eyebrows and the external ear canals. The condition is most common in young babies (cradle cap) and male adults (Schwartz *et al.*, 2006). Seborrhoeic dermatitis generally follows a cyclical course of varying severity throughout adulthood. Causes are unknown but have been linked to the following:

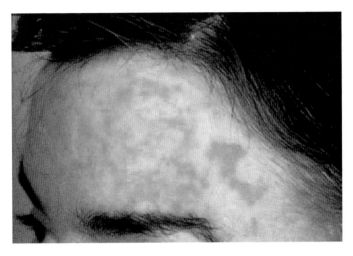

Figure 6.2 Seborrhoeic dermatitis. From Burns T, Breathnach S, Cox N, Griffiths C (2010) *Rook's Textbook of Dermatology*, 8th edn. Reproduced with permission from Wiley-Blackwell.

- Hormonal imbalance (in adults).
- Genetic predisposition.
- Stress.
- Environmental factors.
- Reduced immunity, e.g. HIV.
- Central nervous system disorders (e.g. Parkinson's disease).

(Gupta & Bluhm, 2004)

The most common form of seborrhoeic dermatitis is known as dandruff, a fine, powdery white, itchy scale on the scalp. It may be mistaken for dry skin. Patients may also complain of a burning sensation. If left untreated, the scales may become thick, yellow and greasy and, occasionally, secondary bacterial infection may occur. The severity of the condition often reduces in the summer months.

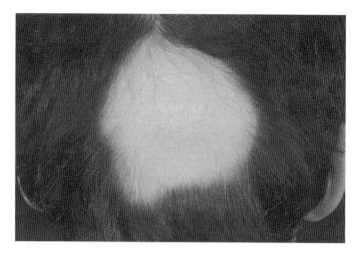

Figure 6.3 Alopecia areata. From Graham-Brown R, Burns T (2007) *Lecture Notes: Dermatology*. Reproduced with permission from Wiley-Blackwell.

Treatment: infants

If scaling is extensive in the scalp of infants, the cradle cap can be softened with oil, gently brushed free with a baby hairbrush and then washed clear with a mild antidandruff shampoo (Sheffield *et al.*, 2007).

General treatment

The use of soap and scrupulous attention to hygiene daily is vital to remove oils from affected areas and improves seborrhoea. Prescribed care includes antifungal preparations and anti-inflammatory agents (e.g. topical steroids). Severe cases may require coal tar for thick scale removal before using steroids. The use of oils such as olive oil can be useful before using a detergent (e.g. washing-up liquid) or coal tar shampoo (Johnson & Nunley, 2000).

Particular care and preparations may be required for different areas of the body. Stubborn scaling of the scalp can be reduced by applying oil with a shower cap overnight before using an antidandruff shampoo in the morning. Care must be taken with some oil preparations and polytar products, which contain arachis (peanut) oil, particularly for people with known nut or soya allergies (British National Formulary, 2009).

Alopecia

Alopecia areata (Figure 6.3) is a chronic inflammatory condition that affects the hair follicles (and less commonly the nails). It affects approximately 0.15% of the UK population (Dobbins *et al.*, 2003) and causes partial hair loss usually on the scalp, eyebrows, eyelashes or beard. The typical pattern is for one or more round bald patches to appear on the scalp (Madani & Shapiro, 2000). Over 50% total loss is viewed as severe (Bolduc & Shapiro, 2001). The condition is reversible, as hair follicles are not destroyed.

Causes

- Genetic disposition: up to 25% of sufferers have a family history.
- Autoimmune disease, e.g. vitiligo, pernicious anaemia and myxoedema (underactive thyroid).
- Possibly a viral infection.
- Possibly stress.

(Madani & Shapiro, 2000; Messenger, 2004)

Autoimmune disease causes the immune system to mistake the affected hair roots (hair follicles) as foreign bodies; mild inflammation leads to hair weakening and falling out (MacDonald Hull *et al.*, 2003). Motivation to socialise or seek employment is reduced, particularly as the condition is unpredictable. Hair recovery may not be complete and there is little indication for the individual as to how long the condition will last or whether it will recur. During recovery, hair will regrow but will be fine and white or grey at first before returning to its normal colour. Without treatment, 80% of people with less than 40% or mild hair loss can expect re-growth within one year as the condition is usually self-limiting (Bolduc and Shapiro, 2001). However, 14–25% of people will deteriorate and present with total scalp or body hair loss.

Treatment

Common treatments, if offered, include steroid treatment either by injection or by topical application. Steroids can be combined with medication for male pattern baldness to stimulate hair growth (MacDonald Hull *et al.*, 2003). Non-medical treatments include counselling to cope with psychological issues, the use of wigs in extreme cases and even dermatology (i.e. the tattooing of eyebrows).

Hair loss associated with chemotherapy

Alopecia as a side effect of cancer treatment is rated the third most distressing symptom after nausea and vomiting (Batchelor, 2001). Hair loss will occur normally 7–10 days after the commencement of chemotherapy and continues for some time after its conclusion. The effects are reversible and around six weeks post-treatment hair growth begins. Cooling the head/scalp during chemotherapy to under 24°C reduces the amount of hair loss. The introduction of cryogel caps (cold caps) has been effective for some patients. However, there has been detection of a slight risk of scalp metastases thought perhaps to be due to the ineffective treatment of seedlings in the scalp owing to the cooling process (Batchelor, 2001).

Hair loss is also a side effect of radiotherapy and the re-growth can take significantly longer. Patients receiving radiotherapy to their head should be advised to continue to wash their hair but they should wash and dry very gently using cooler water than usual with non-perfumed toiletries to avoid skin irritation.

NURSING INTERVENTIONS FOR GENERAL HAIR CARE

Hair should be brushed and/or combed at least daily to keep it healthy and manageable and to prevent matting or tangling.

Brushing removes debris and dirt from the hair and distributes natural hair oils but, if the wrong brush or comb type is used, can cause pain to the scalp and cause abrasions to the cuticle of the hair. When possible, a brush with natural bristles should be used rather than plastic. African people who have naturally curlier and coarser hair should use a wide-toothed comb.

Patients on bed rest will need help from nursing staff to maintain their hair hygiene both through hair dressing (i.e. combing) and/or brushing and washing the hair.

Procedure: Brushing a patient's hair
Equipment

- Brush and/or comb suited to hair type (patient's own or disposable).
- Towel or protective cover.
- Any prescribed treatment for the scalp or hair.
- Hair oils if hair is tangled or matted.

Action	Rationale
Explain each step of any procedure or examination to the patient and gain their consent	Ensures the patient understands the process and encourages their cooperation
Place patient in most appropriate and comfortable position using manual handling techniques and equipment as determined through assessment. Preferably, the patient should be in a sitting position either in a chair or in bed	The patient will be able to tolerate the procedure if comfortable
Decontaminate hands and wear appropriate PPE if there is the presence of infection/infestation or application of prescribed care	Prevents cross-infection
Place a protective cover over the pillow if the patient is in bed or over the shoulders if they are sitting in a chair	Protects the patient/bedding from debris, dirt and shedded hair. Allows assessment for scalp conditions such as seborrhoeic dermatitis (dandruff)
Shake out the hair, removing any styling accessories	
If the hair is very tangled, rub hair oil or 'leave in' conditioner into the ends	Increases ease of brushing/combing and causes less discomfort
Short hair can be brushed/combed at one side of the head and then the other. Longer hair can be parted down the middle and then into manageable sub-sections	Ensures that the complete head of hair is dressed

Continued

Action	Rationale
Taking a small section of the hair, hold the hair near the scalp with one hand and comb or brush through towards the end of the hair with the other	Holding the hair prevents tugging of the scalp
Move methodically over the head until all areas of hair have been brushed or combed	
Restyle the patient's hair according to preference	Promotes individualised care
Clear away equipment following local protocols, noting any debris on the protective cover	Allows assessment for hair conditions such as excessive hair loss or dandruff
Clean brush or comb thoroughly	
Ensure the patient is in a comfortable position and has no further requirements	
Decontaminate hands	
Evaluate and document care, noting whether there is a need for reassessment	Promotes continuity of care

HAIR CLEANSING

Shampoos are detergents designed to remove sebum, sweat, fungal elements, desquamated corneocytes, styling products and dirt. Conditioners moisturise hair to leave the hair soft, smooth, hydrated and low in static (Draelos, 2005). By reducing surface friction, conditioners can also improve the ease of wet and dry combing, which can prevent unwanted hair breakage.

Assessment of the patient must be carried out before washing hair to ensure that the patient does not have any allergies, breathing problems or neck/spinal conditions, which may prevent the patient lying flat.

Some protection and comfort can be given through the use of a shampoo tray or trough to support the neck. Trays are made commercially usually of hard plastic with a U-shaped opening for the neck to rest on. The tray has a tube or a funnel shape that allows water to drain into a bucket. A shampoo trough is a home-made device (Box 6.1).

Box 6.1 Making a shampoo trough

- Roll a towel lengthways into a log.
- Bend the log into a U shape.
- Place the U-shaped towel into a large plastic rubbish bag, maintaining the shape.
- Place the bottom of the U under the person's neck and head. The person's head and hair should rest inside the trough made by the arms of the U.
- Direct the end of the plastic bag to hang over the side of the bed.
- Fold the edges of the plastic bag to form a trough so that the water is channelled into a bucket.

Alternatively – if safety and equipment allow – the bed head can be removed and the bed elevated above the level of a bed trolley. The patient can be assisted using moving and handing equipment (e.g. glide sheets towards the top of the bed). The shoulders and neck remain on the bed but the top of the patient's head overhangs slightly, allowing hair to be washed using a jug and a basin.

Procedure: Hair washing in bed

Assess the patient for dependence levels, moving and handling requirements and what products are normally used. Check whether the patient is prescribed any treatment(s) and arrange for administration by a registered nurse or qualified healthcare assistant. Identify any actual and potential problems in carrying out the procedure and take action to solve or alleviate these with the patient. Do not carry out hair washing if there is any risk to the patient – consider alternatives.

Equipment

- Trolley or bed table.
- Shampoo tray or trough.
- Towels.
- Washcloths/disposable cloth.
- Cotton balls.

- Comb and brush (patient's or disposable).
- Shampoo (patient's or prescribed preparation).
- Hair conditioner if used.
- Plastic bucket or large basin.
- Basin or large jugs with warm water and bath thermometer.
- Plastic jug.
- Protective sheet, e.g. flat continence pad/plastic cape.
- Chair with protective absorbent covering.
- PPE.

Action	Rationale
Explain each step of any procedure or examination to the patient and gain their consent	Ensures the patient understands the process and encourages their cooperation
Assess the patient for ability to lie flat and access a shampoo tray or trough if appropriate	Prevents unnecessary and potentially dangerous strain on the patient's neck
Decontaminate hands and wear a plastic apron	Wet and soiled uniforms are a source of cross-infection. Prevents cross-infection
Ensure privacy and close any windows	Patients who are ill or older risk becoming cold quickly
Prepare the area: place the bucket or large basin on a chair or on the floor with absorbent sheeting underneath	Preparing initially prevents the patient getting cold during the procedure. The receptacle must be lower than the bed to collect used water. Not using absorbent sheeting increases the risk of spills and slips
If not contraindicated through the presence of disease, remove the pillows from under the person's head; lower or remove the bed head	Removing the bed head allows access to the patient and gives the nurse more control during the procedure thus preventing water entering the patient's eyes/ears
Cover the top end of the bed with a waterproof pad to keep the bed from getting wet	This may prevent unnecessary disruption to the patient by having to change bed clothes
Gently lift the patient's head and slide in the shampoo tray with the U opening under the neck. Place a towel underneath the patient's neck for support	Allows used water drainage into a receptacle and prevents spills onto the floor

Action	Rationale
OR	
Using appropriate moving and handling strategies, move the patient towards the top of the bed allowing access to the hair	
Place a towel under the patient's shoulders, bringing it forward towards the chest	Maintains patient comfort
Ensuring the patient can be left safely, fill the jugs or basin with warm water. Check the temperature using a bath thermometer	The correct temperature improves patient comfort and reduces the risk of scalding
Arrange for any prescribed care, e.g. medicated shampoo to be administered. Gather personal toiletries and have them and the basin within reach, e.g. on a trolley	
Check the patient's comfort	
Lower the covers towards the patient's abdomen. It is not necessary to leave the patient's lower half uncovered	This maintains dignity and prevents the patient from becoming cold
Remove the patient's night clothes to prevent dampness from getting wet (pyjama bottoms may be left on). Cover the patient with one or more large towels for privacy and warmth	
Place a warm damp washcloth over the patient's forehead without covering the eyes. If necessary, place cotton balls gently in the ears	A damp washcloth will not slip and the patient's eyes will be protected from soapy water
Fill a jug with warm water from the basin. Carefully wet the patient's hair and make sure the water drains into the bucket or wastebasket	
Apply a small amount of shampoo to the patient's head and gently massage the hair and scalp. Using fresh water, rinse the hair and repeat shampoo if necessary	

Continued

Action	Rationale
Apply conditioner if desired or prescribed and rinse using warm water until the water runs clear (some patients with tangled hair may benefit from having their hair combed while conditioner is still applied)	Soapy residue causes the appearance of soap scum in the hair and the scalp will become irritated and itchy
Gently remove the shampoo tray if in use; squeeze excess water from the hair and gently rub hair dry with a towel	
Remove equipment and return the patient to a comfortable position	Reduces any strain on the patient's neck before combing
Replace any wet linen and assist the patient back into their night clothes	Increases comfort and warmth
Comb or brush the patient's hair into its usual style	Promotes normal living
Use a hairdryer at a cool/warm (not hot) setting if the patient wishes and if the dryer has had all safety checks. Keep moving the hairdryer around the hair, styling in the patient's preferred style	Prevents irritation of the scalp. Prevents the discomfort of prolonged heat on the scalp
Clear away equipment, disposing of linen according to local protocol. Wash and dry all equipment thoroughly, including the patient's brush or comb	Prevents cross-infection
Ensure the patient is comfortable and has no other requirements	
Decontaminate hands	
Document the care and any observations/evaluations made during the procedure	Individualises nursing care

WATERLESS HAIR CARE PRODUCTS

Some patients may not be able to tolerate having their hair washed in bed with water and shampoo. These may be patients who are acutely ill, have skeletal problems, have cognitive deficits or who cannot cooperate throughout the procedure. For some, dry shampoos that can be brushed out are useful, but there is an alternative in the form of a pre-impregnated shampoo cap.

The cap is warmed by following the manufacturer's instructions, placed on the patient's head and the scalp massaged through the cap. The product can then be removed, discarded and the hair styled to the patient's preference.

The procedure releases a conditioning shampoo onto the patient's head that removes dirt, debris and oil. There is no need to rinse and the hair is left 'towel dry' after removal of the cap.

The waterless shampoo cap could be considered too expensive. However, the manufacturers argue that, overall, the cap will actually save money by:

- Improved safety by avoiding using water near electrical equipment.
- Reduces the risk of spills and slips.
- Reduces the moving and handling risk as the cap can be used in any patient position that allows access to the head.
- Laundry bills are reduced.
- Nursing time is reduced.

Infection risk is reduced through the single-use system.

HAIR REMOVAL

Traditionally, hair was removed before surgical procedures to prevent wound infections from stray hairs. However, infection risk was increased through microscopic infected lacerations as a result of using razors (Dougherty & Lister, 2008) and routine removal of hair before surgery is now not recommended (National Institute for Health and Clinical Excellence, 2008). If necessary, hair is removed either the day before surgery using a topical depilatory cream (Dougherty & Lister, 2008) or immediately before surgery using single-use electrical clippers (National Institute for Health and Clinical Excellence, 2008).

Patients may wish to remove body or facial hair for cosmetic reasons. The nurse should try to ensure that the patient is assisted to undertake these procedures. There are, however, certain conditions and treatments where caution is recommended before removing hair. These include patients with very sensitive skin, skin infections (e.g. cellulitis) or when the skin has been traumatised (e.g. sunburn or radiotherapy burns).

Box 6.2 Maintenance of electric shavers

After every use (or at least every third use):

- Remove the cutting head and tap debris into a paper towel.
- Dispose of the debris and towel into a clinical waste bag.
- Some modern shavers may be rinsed out under the tap.

Weekly:

- Brush the cutting foils, taking great care (foils are easily damaged/bent and can cause damage to the skin).
- Remove foils carefully and brush the borders of the cutting blade area.
- Wash and dry the brush thoroughly and return to the box.

Females who have unwanted hair may prefer to use depilatory creams or wax. Depilatory creams can be used in the clinical area but care must be taken to check the patient for sensitivity to the cream before applying it to any great extent. Men may wish their beards and moustaches to be trimmed and should have personal equipment to do so. Hygiene is of importance for men who have beards and moustaches as food and fluid particles can become trapped in the hair. Normal soap and water can be used as part of face washing in most cases.

Shaving is the most convenient and inexpensive way to remove hair, but it can also irritate skin and may have uncomfortable side effects, such as razor burns, in-grown hairs (which if untreated can become infected) and skin dryness. For safety reasons and to promote self-care, individual electric shavers are the preferred option for men while in care. Before an electric shaver can be used, it must be subjected to the statutory checks required by the organisation. However, shavers must never be used communally and need careful maintenance (Box 6.2). Simple cleaning routines (following the manufacturer's instructions) performed on a regular basis prevent the build-up of debris and grease, which interferes with the cutting ability of the razor.

Procedure: Removal of hair using a disposable razor

Assessment includes checking the condition of the skin and that there is no risk to skin health by carrying out the procedure. If the skin is too dry, the risk of razor burns increases. The patient's preferences for toiletries should be ascertained. Ideally, avoid shaving after soaking in a bath as skin swells around the follicles, preventing a close shave. Assess for whether non-sterile gloves are required to prevent possible cross-contamination in the event of bleeding.

Equipment

- Disposable safety razor.
- Shaving foam/cream.
- Pre-shaving preparation (if used), e.g. pre-shave oil.
- Basin of warm water checked using a bath thermometer.
- Table or trolley.
- Towel.
- Protective cape or cover.
- Washcloth/disposable cloth.
- Aftershave balm (if used).
- PPE (apron and gloves).
- Sharps disposal receptacle.

Action	Rationale
Explain each step of any procedure or examination to the patient and gain their consent	Ensures the patient understands the process and encourages their cooperation
Help the patient into a comfortable position that allows the best access to the patient, preferably a chair but this may not be possible	Prevents unnecessary and potentially dangerous strain for the nurse in reaching the patient
Gather all equipment onto a flat surface (table or trolley) within easy reach	Reduces the risk of spills and slips
Cover the patient's shoulders with a protective cape	Maintains patient comfort by preventing water penetrating their clothing
Put on apron, decontaminate hands and put on non-sterile gloves	Prevents cross-infection

Continued

Action	Rationale
Hold a warm face/disposable cloth over the patient's bristles for about 60 seconds or apply pre-shave preparation	Steam and heat opens pores for a closer shave, and wet bristles are softer and easier to cut. Pre-shave oils prepare the skin for a closer shave
Apply shaving foam until the area to be shaved has a thick coverage	Prevents scraping and possible cutting of the skin
Dip the safety razor into the water and then, holding the skin taut, position the razor at a 45° angle to the skin at the top of the beard line on the face	Water prevents the razor snagging on the skin and reduces the risk of cutting the skin
Using a short, firm (but not rough) stroke, draw the razor downwards in the direction of the hair growth	Short strokes prevent the skin being dragged and possibly cut
After each stroke, rinse the razor in the water before making another stroke	As identified above, water prevents snagging
Work logically over the face, from one side of the face towards the centre of the chin and then repeat for the other side. Pay particular attention to the creases at the side of the nose	Ensures all bristles are shaved; older men in particular risk having bristles missed if creases are not pulled taut and shaved
Check that the water is still warm enough for patient comfort and that the covering of shaving foam on the face has not dispersed	Improves the experience for the patient. Too little soap can rub the skin, causing irritation
Continue to shave between the nose and the top lip	
Continue shaving under the chin over the neck area	
When the face has been shaved, remove excess shaving foam with a dry cloth	
Rinse the patient's face thoroughly and pat it dry with a soft towel	Soapy residue causes excess dryness and possible irritation of the skin
Ask the patient to feel the shaved surface and comment as to whether he is content with the shave	Promotes patient-centred care
Apply any aftershave products the patient normally uses, patting on rather than rubbing	Individualises nursing care
Clear away used equipment according to local protocols	Prevents cross-infection and risk of sharps injury

Continued

Action	Rationale
Ensure that the patient is returned to a comfortable position and has no other requirements	
Remove and dispose of PPE	
Document care and evaluation of care in the patient's care plan	Allows the implemented care to be evaluated and identifies possible need for reassessment

New shaving creams have been designed to soothe the skin and prevent drying. Antioxidants and vitamins are to improve skin appearance. Black men in particular may have problems with shaving, as their hair is naturally coarser and may grow back into the skin, causing inflammation and infection.

CONCLUSION

This chapter has highlighted that hair hygiene can be important to a person's feeling of wellbeing. Hair loss, whether permanent or temporary, causes psychological distress, and nurses must carry out care sensitively. The individual nature of a patient's hair type, their grooming preferences and the state of their hair's health all mean that nurses will have to use different approaches if they are to successfully individualise a patient's care.

REFERENCES

Batchelor D (2001) Hair and cancer chemotherapy: Consequences and nursing care: A literature review. *European Journal of Cancer Care* **10**(3): 147–163.

Beom JK, Jung IN, Won SP *et al.* (2006) Hair cuticle differences between Asian and Caucasian females. *International Journal of Dermatology* **45**(12): 1435–1437.

Birch MP, Messenger A (2003) 'Bad hair days': Scalp sebum excretion and the menstrual cycle. *Journal of Cosmetic Dermatology* **2**(3–4): 190–194.

Birch MP, Lashen H, Agarwal S, Messenger AG (2006) Female pattern hair loss: Sebum excretion and the end-organ response to androgens. *British Journal of Dermatology* **154**(1): 85–89.

Bolduc C, Shapiro J (2001) The treatment of alopecia areata. *Dermatologic Therapy* **14**(4): 306–316.

British National Formulary (2009) *British National Formulary*, 58th edn. Pharmaceuticals Press, London.

Chamley CA, Carson P, Randall D *et al.* (2005) *Developmental Anatomy and Physiology of Children*. Elsevier, London.

Dawber R (1996) Hair: Its structure and response to cosmetic preparations. *Clinics in Dermatology* **14**(1): 105–112.

Dawber RPR, Messenger AG (1997) Hair follicle structure, keratinization and the physical properties of hair. In: R Dawber (ed.), *Diseases of the Hair and Scalp*, 3rd edn. Blackwell Science, Oxford, 23–50.

Dobbins HM, Delamere FM, Sladden MJ *et al.* (2003) *Interventions for alopecia areata (Protocol for a Cochrane Review)*. The Cochrane Library. Issue 4. John Wiley & Sons, Ltd, http://www.thecochranelibrary.com, [accessed 16 December 2008].

Dougherty L, Lister SE (eds) (2008) *Royal Marsden Hospital Manual of Clinical Nursing Procedures*, 7th edn. Blackwell Publishing, Oxford.

Draelos ZD (1997) Understanding African-American hair. *Dermatology Nursing* **9**(4): 227–231.

Draelos ZD (2005) *Hair Care: An illustrated dermatologic handbook*. Taylor & Francis, London.

Girman CJ, Rhodes T, Lilly FRW *et al.* (1998) Effects of self-perceived hair loss in a community sample of men. *Dermatology* **197**(3): 223–229.

Gupta AK, Bluhm R (2004) Seborrhoeic dermatitis. *Journal of the European Academy of Dermatology & Venereology* **18**(1): 13–26.

Health Protection Agency (2005) Guidance for the management and control of head lice, http://www.hpa.org.uk/web/HPAwebFile/HPAweb_C/1204100452154, [accessed 10 January 2009].

Johnson BA, Nunley JR (2000) Treatment of seborrhoeic dermatitis. *American Family Physician* **61**(9): 2703–2710.

MacDonald Hull SP, Wood ML, Hutchinson PE *et al.* (2003) Guidelines for the management of alopecia areata. *British Journal of Dermatology* **149**(4): 692–699.

Madani S, Shapiro J (2000) Alopecia areata update. *Journal of the American Academy of Dermatology* **42**(4): 549–566.

McMichael AJ (2007) Hair breakage in normal and weathered hair: Focus on the black patient. *Journal of Investigative Dermatology Symposium Proceedings* **12**: 6–9.

Mehmi M, Abdullah A (2007) The history of hair removal. *British Journal of Dermatology* **157**(suppl. 1): 76–77.

Messenger AG (2004) Alopecia areata. In: T Burns, S Breathnach, N Cox, C Griffiths (eds), *Rook's Textbook of Dermatology*, 7th edn. Blackwell Science, Oxford, 63.36–63.37.

Nash B (2003) Treating head lice: Clinical review. *British Medical Journal* **326**(7401): 1256–1257.

Neinstein LS, Kaufman FR (2002) Abnormal growth and development. In: LS Neinstein (ed.), *Adolescent Health Care*, 4th edn. Lippincott Williams & Wilkins, Philadelphia, 3–51.

Neinstein LS (2004) Medical problems – Dermatology – Hair lesions, http://www.usc.edu/student-affairs/Health_Center/adolhealth/content/b4derm3.html, [accessed 13 October 2009].

National Institute for Health and Clinical Excellence (2008) *Surgical Site Infection: Prevention and treatment of surgical site infection*. Department of Health, London.

Rexbye H, Petersen I, Iachina M *et al.* (2005) Hair loss among elderly men: Etiology and impact on perceived age. *Journal of Gerontology: Medical Sciences* **60A**(8): 1077–1082.

Royal College of General Practitioners (2006) *Sexually Transmitted Infections in Primary Care*. RCGP Sex, Drugs & HIV Task Group. British Association for Sexual Health and HIV, London.

Schwartz RA, Janusz CA, Janniger CK (2006) Seborrheic dermatitis: An overview. *American Family Physician* **74**(1): 125–130.

Scott GR (2001) European guideline for the management of pediculosis pubis. *International Journal of STD & AIDS* **12**(suppl. 3): S62.

Sheffield RC, Crawford P, Wright ST (2007) What's the best treatment for cradle cap? *Journal of Family Practice* **56**(3): 232–233.

Sinclair R, Banfield CC, Dawber RPR (1999) *Handbook of Diseases of the Hair and Scalp*. Blackwell Science, Oxford.

Sinclair RD (2007) Healthy hair: What is it? *Journal of Investigative Dermatology Symposium Proceedings* **12**: 2–5.

Sladden MJ, Johnston GA (2004) Common skin infections in children. *British Medical Journal* **329**(7457): 95–99.

Speare R, Canyon DV (2005) Quantification of blood intake of the head louse: Pediculus humanus capitis. *International Journal of Dermatology* **45**(5): 543–546.

Wendel K, Rompalo A (2002) Scabies and pediculosis pubis: An update of treatment regimens and general review. *Clinical Infectious Diseases* **35**(suppl. 2): S146–S151.

Williams P (1995) An appendage of skin – hair. In: LH Bannister, MM Berry, P Collins *et al.* (eds), *Gray's Anatomy: The anatomical basis of medicine and surgery*, 38th edn. Churchill Livingstone, London, 400–405.

Yang A, Iorizzo M, Vincenzi C *et al.* (2009) Hair extensions: A concerning cause of hair disorders. *British Journal of Dermatology* **160**(1): 207–209.

Methods of Washing

7

THE IMPORTANCE OF WASHING

Having the opportunity to wash meets a person's biopsychosocial needs. Therapeutic bathing alleviates the effects of skin infections and conditions (Ronda & Falce, 2002). The patient feels better as body odour is eliminated and appearance improved, cultural needs are met and washing can induce feelings of comfort and relaxation or stimulation (Sheppard & Brenner, 2000).

Healthcare professionals are faced with meeting the hygiene needs of people with a wide range of physical requirements and cognitive abilities, and all of whom have individual preferences and requirements. Over cleansing of the skin leads to a disruption in the natural balance of the skin flora and can lead to tissue damage (Baranda *et al.*, 2002). Even skin preparations designed for sensitive skin can cause irritation and patients must have care carried out which prevents skin damage (e.g. the use of emollients and protective skin creams).

The aim of this chapter is to help the reader understand how to meet the patient's cleansing needs and the underpinning rationale(s) for care.

LEARNING OUTCOMES

After reading this chapter, the reader will be able to:

❏ Describe the indications for bathing, showering and bed bathing.
❏ Understand the assessment principles behind meeting hygiene needs.
❏ Discuss the evidence base underpinning clinical procedures.

❏ Prepare the patient for the nursing practice.
❏ Collect and prepare the equipment safely.
❏ Carry out the clinical skills relating to personal cleansing.

THE INFLUENCE OF THE LIFESPAN ON BATHING AND SHOWERING

Infancy (0–23 months)

The very young and very old in particular should be bathed with particular care paid to the types of toiletries used. Babies may not require to be bathed daily, as frequent bathing may alter the pH of the skin: topping and tailing, where the baby's face and nappy area are washed, may suffice (Roberts, 2008). Separate water should be used for both, and particular attention must be given to bathing the baby's eyes with sterile water before washing the rest of the face.

Childhood (2–11 years)

Bathing and playing is a normal part of a child's development (Roberts, 2008) and safety is the main concern. Children should not be left alone in the bathroom at any time, although older children may be supervised more discreetly. Parents or the child's carers may be happy to assist with bathing, as this is more familiar for the child. It is important to assess a child's understanding of any restrictions while bathing which their condition may dictate. For example, children with plaster casts would require supervision to ensure that the cast did not get wet.

Adolescence (12–19 years)

Teenagers are more likely to have been brought up having daily showers rather than baths, and this may be their preference. Assessment for safety is required and in clinical areas adolescents can be supervised discreetly, unless there is a cognitive or physical deficit which affects their independence. If assistance is required, the teenager, where possible, should be given the choice of having a family member or a healthcare professional to carry out the care.

Adulthood (20–64 years)

The main issue for adults as well as ensuring safety is to raise awareness of the potential for cross-infection. Most adults are used to daily bathing and/or showering and this has become the norm in our society. When illness or debility means that it may not be possible to bathe daily, it is important that healthcare professionals can recognise the possible feelings of discomfort in patients and take measures to compensate.

Older age (65+ years)

Older people should ideally not be bathed on a daily basis, in order to preserve the pH of their skin and to prevent drying out and possible deterioration. Older people who happen to have a problem with incontinence will require hygiene measures to prevent urine from causing excoriation of the skin. When assisting a patient to choose a continence aid, it should be remembered that to maintain skin health an aid should not be chosen if the urine is going to lie next to the skin rather than being channelled away or absorbed (Hampton, 2004). No-rinse foam can be useful for cleaning the skin of patients with incontinence as it is less irritating and provides a protective barrier over the skin. While personal choice is important regarding the use of toiletries, older people's skin in particular dries out from the effects of highly perfumed soaps.

PATIENTS WITH COGNITIVE PROBLEMS

Patients who have cognitive problems, for example those with dementia or people with profound learning disabilities, may have trouble understanding the intentions of healthcare professionals when undergoing bathing or showering procedures. When this happens, the cognitive problems may be accompanied by behavioural problems such as physical and verbal aggression and wandering (Rasin & Barrick, 2004). Up to 90% of older people with dementia will exhibit agitation on becoming aware that they will be bathed and disturbed behaviours can extend as far as hitting, punching, slapping and pushing (Hoeffer *et al.*, 1997). These symptoms may be attributed to reactions to environmental factors (e.g. lighting noise), the number of carers and the patient's coping mechanisms and functional ability (Kolanowski, 1999).

Remember that people with a learning disability or cognitive impairment may have difficulty processing information, following instructions or understanding what is happening. Try to keep sensory stimuli to a minimum (e.g. avoid clutter or harsh lighting). However, familiar music and a warm room may help as well as the healthcare professional(s) appearing relaxed rather than anticipating trouble.

INDIVIDUALITY IN LIVING (NORMAL LIVING): ASSESSMENT

When encouraging a patient towards independence in meeting hygiene needs, it is important to assess and identify what washing facilities the patient has at home and who (if anyone) will be available to assist. There is little point in encouraging a patient to be independent in showering if there is no shower available on discharge. In order to individualise care, it is important to assess each patient, and this assessment should include:

- Discovering the patient's personal preference, e.g. bath or shower, morning or evening.
- Judging their understanding of and consent to the process.
- Understanding safety concerns, including mobility, equipment required, water temperature.
- Infection control.
- Knowing the patient's physical ability to cope with and contribute to the process.

Physical health and how people live normally and what bathing/showering facilities are available in the home may impact on whether a person prefers bathing, showering, sponge bathing or other methods of meeting hygiene needs (Naik *et al.*, 2004). Older people in particular and those with mental health problems report bathing difficulties due to disease processes and mobility problems (Murphy *et al.*, 2007). The presence of pressure sores can affect the comfort of bathing, where sitting can cause additional pain and discomfort as can fear of the process in

Table 7.1 Advantages/disadvantages of baths and showers

Bathing	Showering
Advantages	*Advantages*
Warmth and comfort: the patient is often more relaxed during bathing compared to showering	Tend to be viewed as more hygienic for cleaning patient after episodes of incontinence
A bath can encourage movement of limbs in comfort	Showers can be invigorating
Accidental slips are less common with bathing	Less water is used
Full access to the patient can usually be facilitated round the bath	Showering tends to be quicker than bathing
Emollients are easier to add to bath water and cause less risk of slips to the patient and nursing staff	
Disadvantages	*Disadvantages*
The procedure often takes longer than for showering which some patients may find more tiring	The splashing from showers can increase the risk of slips for nursing staff and patients
Water may become soiled if the patient is faecally incontinent	Patients tend to get colder when showering compared to bathing
More water is used than for showering	Shower chairs or trolleys can cause moving and handling problems, particularly if the shower space is limited
Bath hoists can cause patients to feel vulnerable when they are raised and moved over the bath	

patients who are unable to understand and cooperate. Alternative methods for meeting hygiene needs should be identified and discussed with the patient, for example simple daily washing.

Aside from patient preference, the decision to bath or shower a patient may be made according to clinical need (Fitzgerald, 2000), and both approaches have advantages and disadvantages (Table 7.1).

FACTORS INFLUENCING MEETING HYGIENE NEEDS
Physical
For patients who are physically frail, options and aids are available (see below) to ensure that any risks to the patient or healthcare professional are managed. Consideration and

assessment must be given not just to the patient's physical ability with regards to such activities of living (ALs) as mobility and breathing but how independent the patient is in other ALs, such as sleeping and expressing sexuality. Patients may be physically able to bath but may be too tired to cope with the procedure. Skin conditions may necessitate washing that is more frequent.

Psychological

Assessment of the patient with cognitive problems is vital to ensure minimum distress for people with difficulty understanding the process. Patients who have a learning disability or those with dementia may not understand why someone who to them is a stranger is removing their clothes and may become agitated or even openly upset. Relatives and carers can be consulted regarding the patient's normal reactions to, and communication of, stressors before trying to bath or shower the patient. This could provide the information for nursing staff to recognise patient reactions to bathwater temperature, too many carers, heat or cold or having their clothes removed (Clark, 2006). Relatives can also describe the patient's normal bathing habits (e.g. bath or shower preference) familiar equipment (e.g. washcloths, soaps and smells), which will be familiar to the patient and may reduce stress. Knowing the patient's normal use of language to describe bathing (e.g. having a sponge bath, 'washing over' or referring to the bath as a 'tub') can also help to familiarise the procedure for the patient.

Some patients are found to be less agitated when undergoing a variation of a bed bath – the thermal bath – as an alternative to conventional bathing (see 'Bed bathing' section) (Kovach and Meyer-Arnold, 1997; Dunn *et al.*, 2002). Men were particularly found to be calmer than women when being bathed (Dunn *et al.*, 2002). Ready-prepared, no-rinse-formulae bag baths are also useful for people with cognitive problems as the procedure is shorter, less complicated and reduces the risk of injury to the patient, for example skin tears (Birch & Coggins, 2003).

Sociocultural

Cultural beliefs and customs may demand or prevent specific interventions, for example some people must only wash in running water and others will prefer family members or same-sex members to carry out the activity (Henley & Schott, 1999).

Patients' reluctance to bath or shower should be explored for underpinning reasons; these may include pain or fear (Nazarko, 2007). Adopting a problem-solving approach and intervening sensitively may address these problems and enhance the patient's quality of life in this area of care. Some religions will dictate that same-sex carers carry out bathing; in these circumstances, providing a risk assessment has been carried out, some people may prefer their own family to meet their hygiene needs rather than a healthcare professional. If patients who would normally wash under running water as part of their belief system need to bathe, a jug can be provided to ensure that the water can still run over them.

ENVIRONMENTAL INFLUENCES ON BATHING AND SHOWERING

The bath/shower room is an area where safety may be compromised in many ways. Before planning how to best meet a person's hygiene needs, a comprehensive moving and handling assessment must be carried out (Switzer, 2001).

The risk of falls and injury can increase through hard surfaces becoming slippery if allowed to remain wet. Non-slip flooring is recommended but not always available; therefore, the use of non-slip mats and extra attention to keeping floors dry and free from spills such as water, soap or talcum powder is important. Non-slip mats should be washed and dried after each bath/ shower according to local infection control policy and replaced frequently. Often bath/shower rooms are small, restricting movement particularly if mobilising equipment is required.

In these circumstances, healthcare staff are also at risk of injury. Bath/shower rooms must be equipped with grab rails and handles which have been placed strategically where the patient can use them to facilitate safe standing/transferring (Swann,

2005). These may be wall-mounted, fixed to the floor or integral to the bath or shower. Occasionally, these aids can impede mobility (i.e. floor-to-ceiling poles can stop equipment being taken right up to the bath or shower). It needs to be remembered that not all aids will be suitable for all people in all circumstances; individual assessment remains vital (Swann, 2005). Bath/shower seats and aids are available for assisting balance while washing.

There are several variations: some may be discrete units that can be used for either the bath or the shower, some attach to the bath when needed and are equipped with harnesses for safety and others have in-built transfer systems. It should be remembered that people may have just as much difficulty getting out of the bath as getting in and this process can put a severe strain on carers' musculoskeletal systems.

BATHING AIDS
Grab rails
These should be coated with a non-slip surface to allow the patient to hold on safely while climbing into the bath (Collins, 2001). They are particularly appropriate for use with step-in baths or when assisting a patient towards independence prior to discharge home. Grab rails can also contribute to ease of exiting a bath – something which is often reported by older people as more difficult than getting in (Jepson & Evans, 2003). Grab rails are only useful if the patient has enough upper-body strength to be able to hold on safely and may, depending on where they are sited, prevent the safe use of hoists.

Bath boards
These boards, which lie across the bath, allow a person to sit on the side and manoeuvre their legs over into the bath and slide across to the middle of the bath. Care must be taken to ensure that the board is properly fixed to the bath sides and that no more than 10 cm hangs over; otherwise, there is a risk of tipping (Jepson & Evans, 2003). Some bath boards are slatted to allow access for washing the buttocks. The patient can sit on the bath board while being dried.

Bath seats

These can be used in conjunction with bath boards – where the patient will lower themselves onto the seat from the board – or independently. Bath seats come in different heights, although lower seats require more effort to exit the bath from a sitting position. Bath seats cannot be used with fibreglass baths as the bath may split under the pressure.

Lifting aids/bath hoists

Equipment to raise the patient over the bath and then lower them into the bathwater comes in a variety of types.

The majority of hoists have a fixed seat which is raised manually or by control pads/hydraulic systems. The size of the seats can sometimes prevent complete lowering to the bottom of the bath and more water is needed for adequate coverage.

Some hoists have slings rather than seats for extremely frail or disabled patients. There needs to be enough room for the patient's bed to be in the bathroom as well as the hoist. The patient will be raised from the bed on the sling and then returned to the bed from the wet sling to be removed and the patient dried and dressed on the bed.

Patients can feel vulnerable and afraid during the process of lowering and rising from the bath. They will need to know exactly what to expect during the process and how they can assist and contribute to the process. They will also need constant reassurance.

Bath cushions

Bath cushions can be used to protect people with bony prominences (e.g. the sacrum) from pressure and discomfort while bathing. They should be made of waterproof material and be heavy enough to stay static during bathing; otherwise, the patient may be at risk of losing their sitting balance while in the bath.

BATH TYPES

Adjustable-height baths

These baths are most often found in hospital environments. The bath can be adjusted to a suitable height to prevent back strain or injury. Another advantage is that adjustable-height baths can accommodate most bath hoists.

Walk-in baths

These have the advantage that people with disabilities can walk straight in and sit during bathing without having climb in or raise the legs, which may increase the risk of falling. Some walk-in baths have a small step to be negotiated before sitting and may be difficult for some people to use. The integral seat can be brought forward to the bath entrance in some models. However, the integral seat in these baths tends to be fairly low and some people may find difficulty rising from the sitting position. Equally, the patient must be seated and the door firmly fixed in place before the bathwater can be run or drained. This can cause the patient to become cold and feel embarrassed during the time taken to fill and empty the bath.

Baths with integral seats

Baths with a seat fixed to the side of the bath which can be turned manually or electronically to take the person from the side of the bath over the bathwater are available. This reduces the need for complicated movements, which may be difficult for some people (Fitzgerald, 2000).

Tilting baths

These baths tilt to allow easier access for the patient. The bath is then righted and filled with water. Again, however, the patient must remain in the bath while it fills and drains.

Baths with side access

Useful for patients who use wheelchairs, these baths require the patient to be able to transfer laterally.

SAFETY

Water temperature presents another potential hazard, particularly for the very young, very old and cognitively impaired. Patients have been scalded and have even died after healthcare workers have failed to monitor the temperature of bathwater, which should be no more than 43°C (NHS Estates, 2007). Many baths and showers are currently available with in-built thermostatic control; however, the responsibility for patients' safety remains with healthcare staff and water temperature should still be checked manually using a bath thermometer before being used by the patient (Switzer, 2001).

More specialist bathing equipment will be required for patients with complex needs or for those who are exceedingly physically and/or cognitively frail.

Accidental ingestion of cleaning fluids or personal toiletries should be avoided by following local procedures for the storage of chemicals.

POLITICO-ECONOMIC INFLUENCES ON MEETING HYGIENE NEEDS

Almost one in 10 patients will develop a hospital-acquired infection (HAI) (Emmerson *et al.*, 1996). The costs of HAI are high to both the patient through increased length of stay, increased fear and increased risk of death for some patients and to the NHS through longer waiting lists and increased care costs and resource use. Poor infection control measures can increase the risk of infection during and after bathing, showering or a bed bath; particularly for pre- and post-operative patients, patients who are immunosuppressed, those patients undergoing chemotherapy, older patients and those with wounds or who are undergoing invasive treatment such as intravenous therapy or have post-operative drains in situ.

Healthcare staff should use personal protective equipment (PPE) as directed by local policies. In the case of personal hygiene, wearing a plastic apron means that the contact surface of the nurse's uniform is non-penetrable by water, blood or body fluids. This cuts the risk of transferring infection from patient to patient, patient to nurse or within different areas within the clinical environment (Dougherty & Lister, 2008).

Thorough cleaning of bath/shower rooms and toilets is vital to prevent cross-infection. Local policy should be used for general hygiene measures with specialist interventions used for patients who have known infections, such as methicillin-resistant *Staphylococcus aureus* (MRSA) or hepatitis B.

Cleaning and effective decontamination and sterilization of all reusable equipment such as hoists, baths and showers is integral to protecting the patient. Each item should be cleaned on the basis of risk assessment for each patient who has used or will require the equipment (Ward, 2001). The nurse has an additional responsibility to ensure that all equipment is in safe working order and maintained according to manufacturers' guidelines (NHS Estates, 2005).

INDIVIDUALISING NURSING CARE

A bath should be treated as a therapeutic part of patient care and not as a chore. There is a habit in some clinical areas to identify a particular day for each patient to be bathed. While this ensures that the patient does receive a regular bath, it takes away the opportunity to offer a bath to a patient at night if they are tired or agitated. Patients are often bathed in the afternoon, because that is when most staff are on duty. However, nurses should ask themselves whether the patient would normally have a bath then (as opposed to first thing in the morning or last thing at night, which are when most people normally have baths).

Privacy and dignity are paramount to carrying out this activity, and intimate care must be carried out with sensitivity. Patients may feel the need to bath alone and to lock the bathroom door, putting themselves at risk of help being delayed should they have an accident. A detailed and extensive risk assessment that incorporates the expertise of the multi-professional team and the wishes of the patient must be carried out. Personal privacy may not be possible and patients will need to be encouraged to accept help with personal hygiene.

To prevent cross-infection, items such as toiletries, towel bales and specialist equipment should not be stored in bathrooms. Each patient should have individual personal toiletries or be provided with disposable toiletries until personal equipment is available.

It is recommended that disposable cloths be used for intimate care of the genitals and then disposed of through clinical waste procedures. Personal cloths, if used, should be rinsed thoroughly, wrung out and hung to dry at the back of the patient's own locker.

The condition of the patient may dictate whether it is advisable to shower or bathe. Pre-operative showering is found to reduce skin flora more effectively than bathing and therefore is more likely to reduce the risk of intra-operative infection.

For all patients who have broken skin, protective dressings should be used while showering or bathing. Extra care is needed for older patients who have skin which is frailer and more likely to break down.

Procedure: Preparing a bathroom safely

It is important that the room be prepared for the patient before the procedure starts. This ensures that the room is safe for use and that the nurse does not have to leave the patient unsupervised to retrieve equipment during the procedure.

Action	Rationale
Ensure that the room temperature is comfortably warm	Prevents patients feeling cold and not enjoying the procedure
Ensure that any radiators in the room are warm (not hot) and covered by radiator guards	Hot radiators increase the risk of burns to people with fragile skin. Radiator covers will protect anybody who falls accidentally against the radiator
Ensure that the bath is clean, dry and ready for use. If it is not, clean according to local infection control policy	Prevents cross-infection from a moist, contaminated source
If the bathwater is thermostatically controlled, ensure that the setting is for no higher than 43°C and lower if appropriate	Prevents the risk of burns to vulnerable skin
Ensure that there is a functioning bath thermometer in the bathroom	Avoids the patient being assisted into bathwater which is too cold or too hot for comfort

Action	Rationale
Ensure that any non-slip mats (for outside or inside the bath) have been thoroughly cleaned and dried. If they haven't been, clean according to local infection control policy	Mats harbour bacteria and must be cleaned effectively after each and every use
Ensure that the floor of the room is dry and free from spillages (e.g. talcum powder or bath foam). If it is not, clean up spills and dry thoroughly	Reduces the risk of injury through accidental slips
Ensure that there is a clean and dry chair in the bathroom for the patient to use	Patients may feel tired while undressing/dressing and may need to sit for part of the procedure. Patients with poor balance can sit while being assisted to dress/undress
Bring towels to the bathroom in preparation for the patient bathing	Towels can be used to cover the patient at any stage and improve dignity. Having towels to hand reduces the need to leave the patient unattended
Clear away any unnecessary obstacles from the bathroom	Aids moving and handling and prevents the patient/nurse accidentally tripping
Ensure that no cleaning solutions are left sitting out. If any are, store them safely out of sight	Young children and patients with cognitive deficits may accidentally ingest liquids
Bring in a receptacle for used linen	Prevents having to leave the patient. Prevents the risk of cross-infection from leaving linen/towels lying on the floor
Ensure that there is a waste bin and a clinical waste bin or have waste bags to hand	Reduces cross-infection by being able to dispose of any soiled dressings, incontinence aids, tissues in waste bins
Ensure that any safety equipment (e.g. grab rails) are clean, dry, secure and in good working order. If they are not, clean according to local infection control policy	Reduces cross-infection and the risk of accidental injury through faulty equipment

Continued

Action	Rationale
Ensure that any moving/handling equipment (e.g. bath hoists) are clean, dry and in good working order; include checks of the brakes and manoeuvrability. Any faults should be reported and the patient's bath delayed until fully functioning equipment is available	Reduces the infection risk. Reduces the risk of injury to the patient or nurse
Ensure that the nurse call system is fully functioning. If it is not, two nurses should be in attendance	The nurse needs to be able to summon help in the event of acute illness/accident
Ensure that there is a hook or clothes hanger for the patient's clothes	Avoids clothing being contaminated from the floor and prevents tripping accidents
Close any windows and blinds/ covers	Preserves patient dignity and adds warmth to the bathroom
Bring the patient's clothes and toiletries to the bathroom and hang clothes	Individualises patient care and allows the nurse to give full attention to assisting the patient to the bathroom without having to carry other articles. Avoids having to leave the patient in order to fetch articles for the patient
Where possible, avoid running the bathwater until the patient is in the bathroom	Reduces the risk of accidental flooding. Reduces the risk of another patient entering the bathwater unseen

Procedure: Bathing a patient

Before bathing any patient, check the moving and handling assessment to identify which aids and how many nursing staff will be required. Check the medicine prescription sheet – or ask the registered nurse to check – and arrange for any prescribed care to be added to the bath or available for patient use. Ensure that the bathroom has been prepared safely (see above). Assess whether the patient needs pain relief before having a bath and time the bath accordingly.

Equipment

Before bringing the patient to the bathroom:

- Patient's toiletries.
- Washcloths.
- Disposable cloths.
- Towels.
- Patient's clean clothing.
- Bath thermometer.
- Prescribed care, e.g. bath additives.
- PPE (apron and gloves).

Action	Rationale
Explain each step of any procedure or examination to the patient and gain their consent	Ensures the patient understands the process and encourages their cooperation
Leave the patient safely in bed or seated, decontaminate hands and prepare the bathroom	Prevents the patient for becoming cold before bathing or being exposed to cross-infection
Check the patient's care plan for any additional care (e.g. eye care, moving and handling requirements, infection control requirements, skin care and prescribed care)	Increases continuity of care
Ascertain the patient's assessed level of independence	Evaluates improvement or deterioration in the patient's condition
On returning to the patient, assist the patient into their dressing robe and ensure they are covered well	Preserves the patient's dignity and prevents them from becoming cold
Ask the patient whether they require to use the toilet facilities before bathing	Increases comfort for the patient during the procedure
Assist the patient to the bathroom either by walking with them or by using the transporting aid identified in the patient's care plan	Reduces the risk of injury
With the patient safely seated on either a chair or the seat part of the bath hoist, begin to run the bathwater to a maximum of 43°C. Run some cold water into the bath first before turning on the hot water tap	Maintains patient safety by reducing the risk of scalding

Continued

Action	Rationale
Add – or arrange to have added – any prescribed bath preparations **OR** Add any toiletries of the patient's choice (consider safety)	Aids individualised and therapeutic care
While the bathwater is running, assist the patient out of their clothes. If hospital issue or for hospital laundry, place in the appropriate soiled-linen receptacle. If patient's own clothes, hang up on a hook or clothes hanger	Saves the bathwater cooling while the patient gets undressed. Prevents cross-infection
While undressing the patient cover them with a towel(s) and/or drape a dressing robe over their shoulders until the bath is ready	Maintains dignity and prevents chilling
Cover any wounds with waterproof dressing(s)	Prevents cross-infection
Check the temperature of the bathwater with the bath thermometer	Increases patient comfort during the procedure and prevents the risk of accidental scalding
Using the moving and handling techniques identified in the patient's care plan, assist them into the bath; reassure the patient of their safety throughout. If a bath hoist is used, ensure that the patient is safely enclosed on the hoist (either by straps or chair arms) and that the brakes are applied when the hoist is in position	Patients can feel vulnerable when entering baths; they require reassurance that they will not fall or be hurt
Discuss with the patient how they can/wish to contribute to the procedure	Increases individualised care
Ask the patient whether they use soap on their face; using a clean (or disposable) washcloth, wash the patient's face, ears and neck **OR** Offer the washcloth to the patient to wash their own face, ears and neck	Individualises patient care
Dry the patient's face, ears and neck **OR** Offer the towel to the patient to dry their face, ears and neck	A wet face becomes itchy and uncomfortable

Action	Rationale
Using a fresh washcloth, encourage the patient to wash themselves with support	Encourages independence in self-care
OR	
Wash the patient's torso, including their back and legs	
Check the patient's skin for abnormalities	Evaluates the effectiveness of previous nursing interventions
Assess/reassess the patient's level of dependence	Evaluates the effectiveness of previous nursing interventions
Wash the patient's feet, paying particular attention to between their toes; check their feet for any abnormalities	Feet are vulnerable to abnormalities that prevent the patient mobilising
Explain to the patient that you are going to wash their genitals using a disposable cloth, and gain consent	
OR	
Offer a disposable washcloth to the patient to wash their genital area	
Dispose of the cloth into a waste disposal bag	Prevents cross-infection
Allow the patient to soak in the bath and take the opportunity to converse with them	Develops the nurse–patient relationship and makes the experience more pleasant for the patient
The patient may appreciate the chance to have their hair washed. If the bath has an integral shower head, this can be used to wash and rinse the patient's hair. Otherwise, use a jug filled from the tap – ensure that the water temperature is safe while filling – always run the cold water tap as well as the hot	Adds to individualised care
When the patient is ready, using the appropriate moving and handling aids, help the patient out of the bath and begin to drain the bathwater	Reduces the risk of injury to the patient and/or the healthcare professional

Continued

Action	Rationale
If the patient is using a bath hoist, the buttocks can be washed through the aperture (opening) of the seat when the patient is raised above the bath; use a fresh disposable washcloth to wash and rinse the buttocks **OR** If the patient is standing, ensure they are balanced and wash and rinse their buttocks before they exit the bath	
Immediately on exiting the bath, cover the patient's shoulders and groin/legs with towels. Begin to dry the patient, patting gently but firmly with the towels	Increases patient dignity and prevents the patient from becoming cold. Overly vigorous rubbing can injure the skin of some patient groups (e.g. older people or people with skin conditions)
Remove any protective covers from wounds and dispose of in a clinical waste bag	Prevents cross-infection
Ensure that the skin is completely dry over the patient's face, arms and upper body; check all skin folds (particularly under the breasts for females)	Prevents cracking or soreness of the skin folds. May prevent fungal infections in skin folds
Apply any prescribed topical care according to the prescription **AND/OR** Apply deodorant, body lotion, talcum powder (sparingly) as the patient wishes	Individualises care and adds to therapeutic care
Dress or assist the patient to dress their upper body	
Dry the feet and legs thoroughly, including skin folds and between the toes, and apply any prescribed care or the patient's preference of toiletries	Feet are vulnerable to fungal foot infections/nail infections if not dried properly
Dry the patient's groin area and genitals thoroughly and apply any prescribed care	Prevents irritation and redness from poorly cared for skin
Dress or assist the patient to dress their lower body	

Action	Rationale
If the patient is able to stand, dry their buttocks, apply any prescribed topical preparations and complete the dressing process **OR** Using a mechanical standing/transferring aid and with the assistance of a second nurse, dry the patient's buttocks, apply any prescribed topical preparations and complete the dressing process	
Rinse the patient's washcloth(s) thoroughly and wring dry, place with the wash bag. **NB:** do not wrap it around the bar of soap	Not rinsing and airing the washcloth, or wrapping it round a cake of soap and not cleaning and drying wash bowls thoroughly after use can create a 'soup' of bacteria, which is then transferred back onto the patient's skin during the next use
The patient may wish to take the opportunity of cleaning their teeth or dentures before returning to their bed (see Chapter 3)	Individualises patient care
Assist the patient back to the bedside either by walking or by using the transporting aid identified in the patient's care plan	Individualises care and reduces the risk of injury
Ensure that the patient is comfortable and safe before returning to the bathroom to clear up	
Wash the bath and all equipment used according to local infection control policies and dry thoroughly using disposable towels	Reduces the risk of cross-infection
Clear away all used linen receptacles, disposable bags	
Ensure that all equipment is in working order	Reduces the risk of injury to the patient or the nurse
Ensure that the floor is clean, dry and free from spills	Reduces the risk of slipping and reduces cross-infection
Remove PPE and decontaminate hands	

Continued

Action	Rationale
Return the patient's clothes and toiletries to them and store safely (used washcloths should be hung over a rail at the back of the patient's locker to dry by airing)	
Check whether the patient has any outstanding care (e.g. eye care, care of hearing aids) and whether they require their hair to be dried and styled. The patient may require to be assisted with shaving (see Chapter 6)	Individualises therapeutic care
Decontaminate hands	Prevents cross-infection
Record care in the patient's care plans, evaluate care and identify any reassessment needed	Aids the nursing process for individualising nursing care

Procedure: Showering a patient

Showering patients may be quicker and safer than bathing, particularly in the patient's own home. Adaptations can be made to showers before discharge (e.g. levers can be added to the shower taps/controls for easier use). Clinical areas may have a variety of shower rooms; some are relatively cramped with just a shower curtain for privacy. Other areas may have wet rooms, where the whole room appears to be a large shower area.

There are now several aids for patients to improve independence and/or safety in the shower areas, which include:

Shower units

- *Level access showers:* the patient does not need to step up into the shower, as the unit is level with the floor. The additional advantage of these showers is that there is good wheeled access to them.
- *Integral seats:* the shower cabinet has a seat attached, which can revolve outside of the cabinet. This aids safer dressing and transfers for the patient and the nurse.
- *Open showers:* these showers are the only equipment (apart from moving and handling aids) within the room. The floor is

set at a slope to allow water to drain safely without increasing the risk of slipping to the patient and the nurse. There should be a shower wall or a shower screen to protect the nurse from becoming over wet during the procedure. The advantage of these rooms is that there is plenty room for moving and handling.

Shower aids

- *Shower trolley:* these are long trolleys with raised but flexible sides upon which very disabled or dependent patients can be showered. The patient would be undressed on their bed and then hoisted onto the trolley (and covered) to be taken to the shower room. They have an integral plug that can allow the water to drain and to help with hair washing. The trolley has the advantage of being safer from a moving and handling perspective as the nurse does not have to bend to reach the patient, plus the patient can be rolled to allow access to their back and buttocks. However, a disadvantage is that the patient may feel extremely exposed and vulnerable or embarrassed lying naked on a plastic trolley.
- *Shower chair:* these chairs are designed with several drainage holes to allow the patient to be showered safely. Some are supplied with wheels and brakes for short transfers into the shower; others are static and the patient has to be assisted into the shower before they can use the chair. These shower chairs are not usually suitable as transferring equipment from the patient's bed side to the shower room and should not be used as such unless identified as safe to do so by the manufacturer. **NB:** commodes are not suitable for use as shower chairs as they will usually have metal components that will eventually rust.
- *Grab rails:* as with grab rails above/beside a bath, the rails should be covered with a strong grip coating that will not become slippery when wet. Some showers are not suitable for grab rails and a safety pole may be needed. However, these sometimes interfere with moving and handling equipment.

Preparing a shower room

The principles are the same as for preparing a bathroom. Instead of checking bath hoists, the nurse may have to check any equipment used to transfer the patient and the shower chair using the same infection control and safety principles. Shower rooms are often smaller than bathrooms and the nurse may have to have a chair outside the shower area on which to keep the patient's clothes.

NB: The procedure is much the same as for bathing a patient. Alterations to the above procedure will include:

Action	Rationale
In addition to an apron, the nurse may require to wear rubber/plastic overshoes	The floor may become wetter than when bathing and the nurse's shoes should be protected to prevent slipping either in the shower area or in the ward area
The shower should be run while undressing the patient	Allows the water to be run to the correct temperature
The temperature of the shower water must be checked before the patient enters. The water may have to be cooler than 43°C	Some, particularly older, patients may feel that shower water is hotter than bathwater
The patient may have to be assisted up a step into the shower; two nurses may be required	Increases safety in moving and handling
Check with the patient on entering the shower that the water temperature is comfortable	
The patient may require to sit on a shower chair	Reduces the risk of falls. Older patients may feel faint in a shower
Soap products may have to be used on the washcloths so it is important that all soap is rinsed off the patient before they exit the shower	
There is a greater risk of slipping; two nurses may be required to assist the patient out of the shower	
From exiting the shower, the procedure is the same as for bathing a patient	

Bathing and showering are effective measures to clean the patient overall. Patient preference is paramount, as is clear assessment for particular patient needs. The wide range of bathing and showering aids available add to patients' and healthcare professionals' safety and there is ample opportunity for the nurse to make bathing or showering a pleasant experience for the patient.

BED BATHING

Patients may not be able to bath or shower at various points in their life and at this stage bathing the patient in bed will be required when they are unable to meet their own hygiene needs through showering, bathing or washing. This can be for a variety of reasons (Box 7.1).

Bed bathing is often viewed as basic care; however, the process is far more complex. Bed bathing allows the nurse to develop a relationship with the patient (Major, 2005), assess/reassess independence levels and take the opportunity to use health promotion strategies (e.g. encouraging independence and educating around hygiene issues).

Box 7.1 Reasons for carrying out bed bathing

- Following major surgery: the patient may be too ill, have technological equipment in place (drains, intravenous infusions) or surgical instructions may prevent specific movement post-operatively (e.g. hip replacement, spinal surgery).
- During acute illness: the patient may be too debilitated, have varying consciousness levels, be too toxic or their condition may prevent them mobilising.
- While unconscious: this is the highest level of dependence and the unconscious patient will require all their care needs to be met.
- Following trauma: the patient may be too weak to wash independently or the effect of trauma on an area of the body may prevent them for doing so.
- 'End of life' care: the patient will be dependent on nursing staff. The nurse has a duty to ensure that all care needs are met.
- When extremely weak or fatigued because of illness or treatment: treatments such as radiotherapy and chemotherapy may render the patient too weak or nauseated to carry out their own hygiene needs.

Not all patients who would benefit from a bed bath are completely dependent and unable to meet any of their hygiene needs. Many patients will manage some aspects of the procedure, from being able to dry their face through to managing to wash completely apart from, for example, their feet or their back. Therefore, it is important to assess the patient's ability and plan with them how, and if, they can contribute to the process.

Planning care

Before carrying out the procedure of bed bathing, the patient, the environment and general principles of care must be taken into account in order to ensure that the experience is comfortable and safe for the patient.

Safety and infection control

Water should not be too hot or cold. Use of a bath thermometer is always recommended to ensure safe temperature. The environment around the patient must be considered and as many obstacles as possible should be removed. Appliances such as bed cages should be removed when it is safe to do so and any IV infusions, wound drains, tubing and in-dwelling urinary catheters (IUCs) should be moved safely during the procedure.

Comfort

Ensure that the temperature of the room is adequate. It may be perceived as warm for the nurse while working but patients may feel the effect of any draughts, so windows should be closed. The patient should be offered toilet facilities before bed bathing (see below for procedure). If the patient can get onto the commode, this is ideal and the bed area can be prepared before the bed bath or made after the procedure while the patient uses the commode. However, male patients may prefer to use a handheld urinal, or female patients a slipper urinal.

Dignity and privacy

The patient may feel vulnerable and exposed during this procedure, so it is vital to preserve their dignity and allay anxiety throughout. Many patients will prefer to wash their own genitals, and this is to be encouraged. Ensure that the patient can manage such aspects as washing the labia (for women) and under the foreskin (for men), including rinsing properly. Cultural, ethnic and religious preferences must be assessed and observed.

Procedure: Providing a bedpan to a bed-fast patient
Equipment

- Bedpan.
- Flat absorbent pad.
- Toilet tissue.
- Hand wipes.
- PPE (gloves and apron).

Action	Rationale
Explain each step of any procedure or examination to the patient and gain their consent	Ensures the patient understands the process and encourages their cooperation
Assess whether any moving and handling equipment/procedures are required and the number of nurses required for those procedures	Ensures a safe procedure for the patient and the nurse
Draw curtains/shut the door and ensure privacy	The procedure can be embarrassing for patients
Decontaminate hands and put on PPE	
Ask the patient to bend their knees and raise their buttocks if possible	
Slide a protective sheet/pad under the patient's buttocks	The sheet/pad will absorb any accidental spillage during the procedure
Ask the patient to repeat the buttock raise and slide the bedpan under the patient	
Ask the patient to confirm that their buttocks are positioned accurately over the bedpan and there is no painful pressure	Poor positioning can lead to spillage and painful pressure
If possible, help the patient to a sitting position/raise the top of the bed or slide additional pillows under the patient's shoulders	A sitting position aids urination and defecation and prevents urine from running down the patient's legs

Continued

Action	Rationale
The patient may request to hold on to the bed rails for security	
Provide the patient with toilet tissue	
If safe to do so, leave the patient to pass urine/faeces, but do not leave the vicinity. Stay within speaking distance of the patient	Some patients feel unable to eliminate in front of others
When the patient has finished, ensure that they have managed to wipe themselves after urinating	
The patient may drop the toilet tissue into the bedpan or you may have to provide a clinical waste bag for the patient to dispose of the tissue	
If the patient is defecating, it may not be possible for them to clean independently	
Ask the patient to raise their buttocks and slide the bedpan out from under the patient, taking care not to spill the contents	
Remove the bedpan to the sluice/toilet area or leave the bedpan on the bed (on the bottom sheet) but safely away from the patient	
Ask/help the patient to roll on to their side and wipe the buttocks clean of faecal matter. Wipe from the top of the buttocks towards the anus	Wiping towards the anus prevents faecal matter being spread upwards, which can contaminate the patient's clothing or the bed sheets. Faecal matter can cause irritation to the skin if not cleaned away properly
While the patient is on their side, roll the protective sheet towards their body. Ask them to roll over to the other side and slide the protective sheet out from under	
Place the protective sheet in a clinical waste bag (if disposable) or used-linen receptacle if washable	
Offer the patient hand wipes or hand-washing facilities	Increases patient comfort and prevents cross-infection

Action	Rationale
Ensure the patient is comfortable and has access to the nurse call system	Patients who require bedpans are normally bed-fast and therefore will have no other method of attracting a nurse's attention
Return to the bedpan and measure or note contents according to care plan before disposing of the contents into the correct facilities (e.g. toilet pan or sluice)	
Place a disposable bedpan into the macerator or wash according to the machine available	
If reusable, ensure the bedpan is dry and return it to the appropriate storage facility	
Remove PPE and decontaminate hands	Prevents cross-infection
Record elimination output in the patient's documentation, evaluate care and identify any reassessment required	Documentation of elimination allows clear evaluation of the patient's condition, the effect of any prescribed interventions and nursing care. Accurate recording also prevents unnecessary intervention, such as the prescription of laxatives

Procedure: Bed bathing

Poor infection control measures can increase the risk of infection during and after a bed bath. Practices such as failing to change the water frequently when bed bathing can result in an increase of bacteria on the patient's skin as well as being uncomfortable cold. Not rinsing and airing the washcloth if reusable causes the growth of bacteria, which will then be transferred onto the patient's skin during its next use. Wrapping a cloth round a wet cake of soap or not cleaning and drying wash bowls thoroughly cause the same conditions. Basins should be stored upside-down or facing inwards to prevent general dirt and debris from being introduced to the bowl and transferred to the patient's skin during the washing procedure.

Equipment

- Basin of hot water (35–43°C).
- Patient's preference for cleansing (soap or shower gel etc.) or prescribed cleansing agent.
- Patient's toiletries.
- Clean towels.
- Washcloths/disposable cloths.
- Hair care equipment.
- Nail care equipment.
- Clean nightclothes.
- Clean bed linen.
- Trolley or adequate surface.
- Equipment required for clinical skills, e.g. skin care, mouth care, eye care etc.
- Separate receptacles for patient's used/soiled nightclothes, used/soiled bed linen and disposable items.
- PPE.

Action	Rationale
Explain each step of any procedure or examination to the patient and gain their consent	Ensures the patient understands the process and encourages their cooperation
Assess whether any procedures should be carried out before commencing the bed bath (e.g. eye care, oral hygiene)	
Carry out these procedures according to need or patient preference	Individualises nursing care: some patients prefer their teeth to be cleaned before washing
Collect and prepare the equipment ensuring space around bed is adequate for easy access and movement	Ensures that all equipment is available, working and ready for use. Avoids having to leave your patient unnecessarily
Ensure privacy	Reduces patient anxiety and increases dignity
Put on apron and decontaminate hands	Prevents cross-infection
Fill basin with warm water and check the water temperature with a water thermometer	Too cold and the procedure is uncomfortable, too hot and the patient risks being scalded

Action	Rationale
Ensure basin is at least half-full but can be carried easily without risk of spills. Place basin on a flat surface within easy reach of the patient	Too little water gets cold easily and may become too soapy for effective rinsing. Too much water increases the risk of slips and accidents
Add any prescribed preparation(s) (e.g. emollients) to the water or ask a registered nurse to do this for you	Adheres to safe medicine administration procedures
Adjust bed height to appropriate working height and ensure bed brakes are applied. Lower bed rails if appropriate	Protects patient and person from injury
Help the patient into a comfortable position, removing any excess bed linen and appliances (e.g. bed cradle) but leaving patient covered	Allows easy access to the patient while preserving dignity and preventing the patient from being too cold
Assess the patient's continence status and remove any soiled bed linen, replacing with towels for the patient to lie on (see section on bed making in Chapter 8 for disposal of linen)	Prevents contamination of the surrounding skin or water from urine and faeces. Providing something to lie on protects the patient's skin from sticking to the mattress
Assist your patient to remove nightclothes (two-piece night attire, e.g. pyjama tops, can be removed and bottoms left on until needed)	This can be tiring to do when feeling unwell. The patient feels as though modesty is being considered
Recheck water temperature and ask the patient if the water temperature is comfortable	Ensures that the procedure is comfortable for the patient
Check with the patient whether soap or plain water is preferred for face cleaning	Individualises patient care
Using a clean facecloth or a disposable cloth wash, rinse and dry your patient's face, neck and ears, encouraging the patient to assist if possible	Adheres to infection control measures and encourages the patient's independence
Soap should be kept in the soap dish and not the wash bowl during the procedure	Soap kept in the water becomes soft and prone to contamination between washes. The washing water will become too soapy to rinse effectively

Continued

259

Action	Rationale
Wash the patient's hands or allow the patient to wash their own hands. Dry thoroughly	Hands are often contaminated and should be washed before the limbs. Encourages independence in care
It the patient's hands are soiled with urine or faeces, change the water, thoroughly cleaning or changing the basin	Reduces contamination risk
When washing, wash towards any source of infection, e.g. from wrist to armpit and from foot and ankle towards the groin	Reduces the risk of bacteria spreading over the skin surface, washing from extremities towards the centre of the body also increases circulation
When possible, use disposable cloths. Ensure that any cloth is changed when soiled	Reduces the risk of bacteria spreading over the skin surface
Exposing only the part of the body being washed, wash, rinse and dry your patient's arms, chest (particularly under the breasts) and abdomen, back and legs in the order that suits the patient or is required for infection control	Your patient may have a particular preference. Any infected areas should be dealt with last to prevent risk of infection to other areas. Drying thoroughly prevents skin macerating and reduces the risk of fungal infection and excoriated areas
If the top half of the patient is washed front and back, the patient can be assisted back into nightclothes. Take care with nightdresses that they do not get wet from the rest of the procedure	Increases sense of privacy and dignity
Check and change the water regularly to prevent using cold water and to reduce a build-up of soap residue. Ensure temperature is checked before use	Maintains your patient's comfort and prevents the drying effects of soap to the skin
Inform the patient that the genital and buttock area is to be washed and gain permission	
Wash the buttocks, starting from one hip and work towards the cleft of the buttocks. Repeat from the other hip. Using a clean disposable cloth for both washing and rinsing, wash, rinse and thoroughly dry the cleft of the buttocks, working towards the anus	Reduces the risk of spreading faecal flora over the skin

Action	Rationale
Perineal (genital) care can be carried out last. The patient may be able to manage this aspect of care independently. Ensure that perineal washing is from a front-to-back direction, always going towards the anus (including if your patient is undertaking this aspect of cleansing). See 'Perineal care for a dependent patient' section	Reduces the risk of spreading normal perineal skin flora to other areas. Prevents skin flora from the anal areas being spread towards other areas of the perineum
If safe, apply additional toiletries (e.g. body lotion, deodorant and perfume) **OR** If prescribed, apply any prescribed topical preparations	Individualises patient care
Carry out any additional clinical skills required as part of your patient's care	Your patient will require hair care, ear care, eye care and may require skin care, catheter care etc.
If appropriate at this stage, assist your patient into the remainder of their clean nightclothes	To prevent further exertion from the procedure
Make the bed (see Chapter 8) may be done according to patient need (e.g. bed may need to be made first if sheets are wet and/or soiled or your patient may be feeling exposed or cold)	Promoting care according to the individual's needs
Replace equipment and accessories and rearrange furniture round the bed (e.g. bed tables, buzzer etc.). Ensure the patient can reach everything required	Gives the patient control of their environment and access to nursing staff through nurse call system
Ensure your patient is comfortable and has no further needs at this time	Maintains good-quality care
Dispose of all equipment safely and adhere to infection control issues	Prevents cross-infection
Decontaminate your hands	Prevents cross-infection
Document the procedure noting any progress and abnormal findings	To aid communication between colleagues and to monitor the patient's progress

PERINEAL CARE FOR A DEPENDENT PATIENT

The groin area and the genitals need special attention because of the increased risk of infection and the multitude of bacteria which colonise this area. Perineal care can be carried out independently from bed bathing if the patient is incontinent of urine and/or faeces or if the patient has prescribed care, for example prior to the insertion of pessaries. This can be highly embarrassing for the patient and must be carried out with clear explanations and sensitivity. Assessment of the perineal area includes:

- Evidence of redness, irritation or swelling.
- The patient complains of pain or discomfort.
- Evidence of an abnormal discharge or offensive odour.
- The presence of an in-dwelling urinary catheter.
- Recent surgery or childbirth.
- Prescribed care: time of prescription and method of administration.

Patients when possible will prefer to carry out personal care of the genital area independently; however, as part of the assessment process the nurse must determine that they are able to undertake this effectively. Similar to the hygiene principles of washing towards the most contaminated area, cleansing begins with washing and rinsing the groin in a front-to-back motion.

Procedure: Female perineal care
Equipment

- Trolley.
- Towel.
- Disposable washcloths.
- Clinical waste bag.
- Mild soap.
- Basin with warm water and a bath thermometer.
- PPE (non-sterile gloves and apron).

Action	Rationale
Explain each step of any procedure or examination to the patient and gain their consent	Ensures the patient understands the process and encourages their cooperation
Collect and prepare the equipment ensuring space around bed is adequate for easy access and movement	Ensures all equipment is available, working and ready for use. Avoids having to leave your patient unnecessarily
Decontaminate hands and put on PPE	
Fold the bed linen back from the bottom of the bed up to the patient's waist	This stops the patient feeling cold and the patient feels less exposed
Remove the patient's underwear, pyjama bottoms and any incontinence pad (if worn) and cover their genitals with a towel	
Place a towel under the patient's buttocks	Protects the bottom sheet from becoming wet, uncomfortable and contributing to friction or shearing force pressure areas
Using correct moving and handling technique, assist the patient onto their back, ask them to place their heels together and allow their knees to flop apart	
Using the corner of a fresh disposable washcloth with a small amount of mild soap, wipe one side of the outer labia (vagina lips) from front to back; change corners and wipe the other side the same way	Using all four corners prevents the overuse of resources; prevents the over use of soap by adding more soap each wipe
Change corners and, using the fingers of the non-dominant hand, separate the outer labia and wipe one side of the inner labia from front to back and repeat using the last corner of the disposable cloth	
Dispose of the cloth into a clinical waste bag	
Rinse thoroughly in the same manner	

Continued

Action	Rationale
Use either a soft towel or a dry disposable washcloth and gently dry the perineal area	
Apply any prescribed preparation(s)	
Assist the patient into either underwear, continence aids or replace nightwear	
Assist the patient back into a comfortable position with access to the nurse call system	
Clear away all used equipment and dispose of according to local policy	
Remove PPE, decontaminate hands and replace PPE in readiness to wash the basin	Washing the basin using contaminated PPE may prevent effective cleaning
Wash the basin thoroughly using hot water and detergent. Rinse and dry thoroughly	Eliminates the risk of contamination
Store according to local policy, ensuring that the bowl faces inwards	Prevents the introduction of dirt into the bowl
Document care; evaluate the effectives of nursing interventions and identify any areas for reassessment	Ensures continuity of care

Male care

The procedure is similar to that required for a female. A male patient's knees should still be flopped sideways to allow assessment of the scrotum. The nurse should check that the skin is intact and that there is no swelling or discoloration.

The foreskin of the penis should be retracted (pulled back) and the area underneath washed and rinsed gently. The nurse should use a fresh disposable cloth and sweep round the tip of the penis in one direction.

The foreskin should be returned to place and the shaft of the penis washed from tip towards the base of the penis. The penis should then be rinsed and thoroughly dried.

The scrotum should be washed in the direction from the base of the penis down towards the anus. Nurses must consider the potential for embarrassment for the male patient and remain professional.

Firm (not rough) handling may prevent unintentional arousal. However, should a patient become aroused, the nurse can (providing the patient is safe) make an excuse to leave for a short while until the patient is no longer in an aroused state.

Nursing staff should also be aware that conditions such as dementia and certain head injury can mean that the patient may both mistake the circumstances of care and become aroused or may not have control of the circumstances. If this is the case, the patient should not be made to feel ashamed or humiliated.

Alternatives to the traditional bed bath

New technology in hygiene has introduced an alternative to the traditional soap and water bed bath.

For some patients who have fragile skin, for example the older person or an unconscious patient, soap and water can have a detrimental effect on the skin. Although soap makes the removal of dirt and sweat easier than water alone, using soap bars or liquid soap can alter the pH of the skin and strip the skin of its natural oils (Collins & Hampton, 2003). Using a system known as bag bath eliminates the need for water, soap products and even towels (which can harbour bacteria if kept at the locker side). Bag bath is non-perfumed, has Vitamin E and B5 to protect and heal the skin plus a non-ionic skin cleanser. There is an argument that bag bath is an expensive option but Collins and Hampton (2003) argue that the amount of steps involved in the procedure and the equipment involved in traditional bed bathing can be uncomfortable or tiring for the patient as well as a drain on nursing time.

Procedure: Bag bathing
Equipment

- Packet of bag bath (prepared).
- Cover for the patient.
- Hair care equipment.
- Nail care equipment.
- Clean nightclothes.
- Clean bed linen.

- Trolley or adequate surface.
- Equipment required for clinical skills, e.g. skin care, mouth care, eye care etc.
- Separate receptacles for patient's used/soiled nightclothes, used/soiled bed linen and disposable items.
- Clinical waste bag.
- PPE.

Action	Rationale
Explain each step of any procedure or examination to the patient and gain their consent	Ensures the patient understands the process and encourages their cooperation
Assess whether any procedures should be carried out before commencing the bed bath (e.g. eye care, oral hygiene)	
Assess whether any areas of the body are contaminated (e.g. the hands or buttocks may have faecal matter) and need to be washed prior to the procedure	Hands which are contaminated may need to be washed to be socially clean. Using bag bath cloths may spread any faecal contamination over other parts of the body
Prepare and heat the bag bath according to the manufacturer's instructions	Ensures safety of the procedure and prevents over heating of the cloths
Using a pre-moistened bag bath cloth, check temperature comfort of the cloth with the patient and wash the patient's face **OR** Offer the cloth to the patient to wash their own face. Dispose of the cloth in the clinical waste bag	
Using a clean cloth and starting at the patient's side furthest from the nurse, wash the patient's chest, abdomen, arm, hand and axilla. Dispose of the cloth	Ensures that the nurse does not lean over the cleaned part of the patient's body to continue the process
Using a clean cloth, repeat for the patient's side nearest the nurse. Dispose of the cloth	
Using a clean cloth and following the same principle as bed bathing, wash the foot and leg of the patient at the side furthest away. Dispose of the cloth	

Action	Rationale
Repeat for the other foot and leg	
Using correct moving and handling techniques, assist the patient round to lie on their side and wash their back, starting at the neck and finishing having washed their buttocks. Dispose of the cloth	
Assist the patient to lie on their back and with a clean cloth wash their genitals (see above procedure for positioning and the use of a single cloth). Dispose of the cloth	
Assist the patient to dress and continue with bed making and care as for a traditional bed bath	

CARE OF A URINARY CATHETER

Some patients may require an in-dwelling urinary catheter (IUC) at some stage in their treatment. An IUC is passed through the urethra into the bladder and anchored with a balloon inflated with liquid; urine drains through tubing attached to the IUC into a drainage bag (Lockwood *et al.*, 2004) or is blocked by a valve until the patient can release urine into a toilet. There are several reasons why an IUC may be chosen as an appropriate intervention. Some people may choose supra-pubic catheterisation as an alternative to IUC for long-term use (Wagg & Malone-Lee, 1998; Pomfret, 2004). This involves the insertion of a urinary catheter into the bladder through an incision in the anterior abdominal wall. Hygiene in this case requires the nurse to be vigilant in checking that there are no areas of irritation and that no additional treatment is required other than washing, rinsing and drying.

There is a very high risk of catheter-acquired urinary tract infection (CAUTI) particularly with IUCs and so hygiene is extremely important. Standard perineal care as part of a normal personal hygiene regime has been found to be as effective in preventing UTI as the routine use of prescribed antibiotic preparations (Lockwood *et al.*, 2004). The use of normal tap water to meet hygiene needs is as effective as complicated interventions

(Carapeti *et al.*, 1996), although care should be taken that the area does not become irritated when using soap products.

However, as well as the risk of infection passing from the anal and groin area, infection may ascend (travel up) towards the bladder via the IUC if the drainage system is broken. Care to avoid contamination of the catheter bag during personal hygiene is vital. Correct repositioning of the drainage bag after carrying out hygiene is required to ensure efficient drainage of urine from the bladder into the drainage system:

- If the bag is left too high, e.g. left lying on the bed, there is a risk of urine flowing back up the tubing into the urinary tract, with an associated risk of infection.
- If the bag is left too low, e.g. left lying on the floor, there is a danger of traction (pulling) on the catheter, which may cause discomfort or trauma to the patient.
- If more that 30 cm below bladder level, it may cause negative pressure resulting in part of the bladder lining being sucked into the hole at the tip of the catheter, thus causing trauma and blockage.

(Lowthian, 1998)

Where possible, catheter stands should be used to hang bags; drainage bags should NEVER be left lying on the floor, because of the risk of contaminating the bag exterior and drainage tap or kinking of the drainage tubing.

Changing the catheter bag is also part of the hygiene process. It is necessary to change the drainage bag at least weekly or:

- If it is damaged/leaking/soiled.
- If there is an accumulation of sediment present.
- If the catheter is changed.
- If the catheter/drainage bag is accidentally disconnected.

Procedure: Changing a drainage bag (sterile procedure)
Equipment

- Trolley (decontaminated according to local policy).
- Alcohol-impregnated wipes (alco-wipes).

- Container for urine.
- Clinical waste bag.
- Catheter bag in sterile packaging.
- PPE (apron and gloves; some authorities include protective eyewear).

Action	Rationale
Explain each step of any procedure or examination to the patient and gain their consent	Ensures the patient understands the process and encourages their cooperation
Identify when the drainage bag was last changed. Assess whether it is appropriate to change the catheter bag and identify which type of bag should be used as a replacement (e.g. leg bag, night bag)	
Collect and prepare the equipment, ensuring space around bed is adequate for easy access and movement	All equipment is available, working and ready for use. Avoids having to leave your patient unnecessarily
Ensure privacy	To reduce anxiety
Decontaminate hands; put on PPE	Prevents cross-infection
Prepare trolley:	Ensures that the contents are sterile
• Check use-by-date on drainage bag packaging.	
• Check that packaging is intact.	
• Open package and drop urine drainage bag onto the trolley surface.	
Drain any urine in the bag into a suitable container, noting the volume	Reduces the chance of urine spillage/contamination and measures urine for evaluation of care
Dispose of urine according to local policy	
Decontaminate hands and change PPE	Reduces the risk of contamination of urine
Expose catheter/drainage bag junction	
Clean around the junction of the catheter and the bag with an alco-wipe and allow to dry for 30 seconds	Too short a waiting time reduces the effectiveness of the wipe

Continued

Action	Rationale
Hold the urinary catheter in your non-dominant hand without tugging, take hold of the neck of the catheter bag with your other hand, pulling gently, disconnect and place the used catheter bag into the clinical waste bag. Avoid your glove coming into contact with the open end of the catheter	Reduces the risk of contamination by urine onto gloves. Holding the catheter reduces the risk of pulling trauma to the urethra. Reduces cross-contamination from urine to the clean catheter bag
Lift the fresh catheter bag using your non-dominant hand and slide off the protective sheath. Check that the valve for emptying the catheter bag is empty. Transfer to the other hand and connect the new drainage bag by holding the urinary catheter and gently inserting the bag into the catheter up to the hilt	Maintains infection control. Prevents accidental urine spillage onto the linen or floor
Hang the drainage bag on a catheter stand and ensure that the urine is draining	Ensures optimum drainage of urine into the catheter bag
Remove PPE and used equipment, placing into clinical waste bag	Reduces infection risk
Dispose of clinical waste bag according to local policy and decontaminate the trolley	
Decontaminate hands	Prevents cross-infection
Make sure the patient is comfortable, has access to the nurse call system and ensure no further care is required at this time	
Record urine output and document change of bag in the patient's notes	

Any additional care measures that the patient requires should be acted on as part of the hygiene process. The patient may require to be shaved, have oral hygiene needs met and wound dressings attended to. Non-registered nurses may be required to refer to registered nurses for guidance as to the required procedures.

CONCLUSION

This chapter has discussed a range of methods for washing the patient. Meeting cleansing needs contributes to the health and well-being of the patient. Assessments of the patient's preferences and capabilities are important in order to carry out the procedures safely and comfortably. The dignity and comfort of the patient are paramount concerns when carrying out the procedures effectively.

REFERENCES

Baranda L, Gonzales-Amaro R, Torres-Alvares B *et al.* (2002) Correlation between pH and irritant effect of cleansers marketed for dry skin. *International Journal of Dermatology* **41**(8): 494–499.

Birch S, Coggins T (2003) No rinse, one-step bed bath: The effects on the occurrence of skin tears in a long-term care setting. *Ostomy and Wound Management* **49**(1): 64–67.

Carapeti EA, Andrews SM, Bently PG (1996) Randomised study of sterile versus non-sterile urethral catheterization. *Annals of Royal College of Surgeons of England* **78**(1): 59–60.

Collins F (2001) Choosing bathing, showering and toileting equipment. *Nursing & Residential Care* **3**(10): 488–489.

Collins F, Hampton S (2003) BagBath R, the value of simplistic care in the community. *British Journal of Community Nursing* **8**(10): 470–475.

Clark J (2006) Providing intimate care: The views and values of carers. *Learning Disability Practice* **9**(3): 10–15.

Dougherty L, Lister SE (eds) (2008) *Royal Marsden Hospital Manual of Clinical Nursing Procedures*, 7th edn. Blackwell Publishing, Oxford.

Dunn JC, Thiru-Chelvam B, Beck CH (2002) Bathing: Pleasure or pain? *Journal of Gerontological Nursing* **28**(11): 6–13.

Emmerson AM, Enstone JE, Griffin A *et al.* (1996) The second national prevalence survey of infection in hospital: An overview of the results. *Journal of Hospital Infection* **32**(3): 175–190.

Fitzgerald J (2000) Update on bathing solutions. *Nursing & Residential Care* **2**(6): 269–276.

Hampton S (2004) Promoting good hygiene among older residents. *Nursing & Residential Care* **6**(4): 172–176.

Henley A, Schott J (1999) *Culture, Religion and Patient Care in a Multi-ethnic Society*. Age Concern, London.

Hoeffer B, Rader J, McKenzie D *et al.* (1997) Reducing aggressive behavior during bathing cognitively impaired nursing home residents. *Journal of Gerontological Nursing* **23**(5): 16–23.

Jepson J, Evans MJ (2003) Using equipment to solve residents' bathing problems. *Nursing & Residential Care* **5**(10): 466–469.

Kolanowski AM (1999) An overview of the need-driven dementia-compromised behavior model. *Journal of Gerontological Nursing* **25**(9): 7–9.

Kovach CR, Meyer-Arnold EA (1997) Preventing agitated behaviors during bath time. *Geriatric Nursing* **18**(3): 112–114.

Lockwood C, Page T, Conroy-Hiller T, Florence Z (2004) Management of short-term indwelling urethral catheters to prevent urinary tract infections. *JBI Reports* **2**(8): 271–91.

Lowthian P (1998) The dangers of long-term catheter drainage. *British Journal of Nursing* **7**(7), 366–379.

Major C (2005) Meeting hygiene needs. In: L Baillie (ed.), *Developing Practical Nursing Skills*, 2nd edn. Hodder Arnold, London, 236–276.

Murphy SL, Gretebeck KA, Alexander NB (2007) The bath environment, the bathing task, and the older adult: A review and future directions for bathing disability research. *Disability and Rehabilitation* **29**(14): 1067–1075.

Naik AD, Concato J, Gill TM (2004) Bathing disability in community-living older persons: Common, consequential and complex. *Journal of the American Geriatrics Society* **52**(11): 1805–1810.

Nazarko L (2007) Bathing patients with care and dignity. *British Journal of Healthcare Assistants* **1**(2): 73–76.

NHS Estates (2005) 01: Reporting defects and failures and disseminating NHS Estates alerts, http://www.dh.gov.uk/en/ Publicationsandstatistics/Lettersandcirculars/Estatesalerts/ DH_4119176, [accessed 15 October 2009].

NHS Estates (2007) *Safe Bathing: Hot water and surface temperature policy.* NHSE, London.

Pomfret I (2004) Intermittent and indwelling catheterization: A guide. *Nursing & Residential Care* **6**(9): 430, 432, 434.

Rasin J, Barrick AL (2004) Bathing patients with dementia: Concentrating on the patient's needs rather than merely the task. *American Journal of Nursing* **104**(3): 30–32.

Roberts S (2008) Meeting the personal hygiene needs of a hospitalized child. *British Journal of Healthcare Assistants* **2**(5): 214–216.

Ronda L, Falce C (2002) Skin care principles in treating older people. *Primary Health Care* **12**(7): 51–57.

Sheppard C, Brenner PS (2000) The effects of bathing and skin care practices on skin quality and satisfaction with an innovative product. *Journal of Gerontological Nursing* **26**(10): 36–45.

Swann J (2005) Enabling residents to enjoy showering. *Nursing & Residential Care* **7**(11): 516–518.

Switzer J (2001) Supervise a general bath. *Nursing & Residential Care* **3**(5): 226–228.

Wagg A, Malone-Lee J (1998) The management of urinary incontinence in the elderly. *British Journal of Urology* **82**(suppl. 1): 11–17.

Ward B (2001) Infection control policies in nursing homes. *Nursing Standard* **15**(46): 40–44.

Skin Care

8

INTRODUCTION

The skin is the largest organ of the body and one of the most important. Its complex structure provides many protective functions for the internal anatomy of the body (Box 8.1).

The aim of this chapter is to help the reader understand how to meet the patient's cleansing needs and the underpinning rationale(s).

LEARNING OUTCOMES

After reading this chapter, the reader will be able to:

❏ Describe the anatomy and physiology of the skin.
❏ Identify common diseases of the skin during assessment.
❏ Discuss the evidence base underpinning clinical procedures.
❏ Prepare and make beds for patient comfort.
❏ Describe how to position patients safely in bed for comfort;

ANATOMY OF THE SKIN (THE CUTANEOUS MEMBRANE)

Every square inch of skin contains millions of cells and hundreds of sweat glands, oil (sebaceous) glands, blood vessels and nerve endings. Skin is made up of three layers: the **epidermis**, **dermis** and the **subcutaneous tissue** (Thibodeau & Patton, 2008) (Figure 8.1).

The epidermis is the topmost layer of the skin that, although relatively thin, acts as the tough, protective outer layer. The cells of the epidermis are constantly shedding (exfoliating) and renewing. The cycle of replacing all cells takes around one

---

Box 8.1 Protective function of the skin

A healthy, intact skin fulfils the following purposes in order to protect the internal organs from infections and exposure to harmful substances:

- The maintenance of a physical barrier against the external environment, e.g. trauma, toxins and ultraviolet rays.
- Skin structure includes sebum which is acidic and protects against infiltration by bacteria.
- The prevention of fluid loss, such as water and blood.
- Immunologic protection.
- Temperature regulation through sweat production and changes in blood vessel size.
- Pain receptors act as protection against danger.
- Formation of Vitamin D.

(*Source:* Cooper *et al.*, 2005; Watkins, 2008)

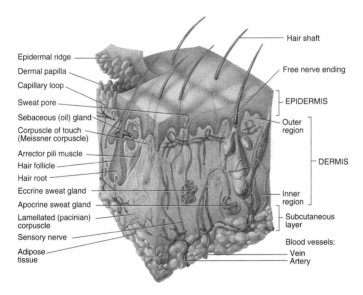

Sectional view of skin and subcutaneous layer

Figure 8.1 Anatomy of the skin. From Tortora GJ, Grabowski SR (2004) *Introduction to the Human Body: Essentials of Anatomy & Physiology*, 6th edn. Reproduced with permission from Wiley-Blackwell.

month; hence skin as an organ can regenerate, which allows effective healing.

The epidermis itself comprises many layers; the cells of the innermost layer, reproduce constantly. As the new cells regenerate, they push other new cells towards the skin's surface through the other epidermal layers (strata). On reaching the outer epidermal layer, they are filled with the protein **keratin**. Keratin is waterproof and hard-wearing. It is a basic component of hair, skin, nails and acts as a barrier.

The tightly packed cells deep in the epidermis are **melanocytes**, which production melanin, the pigment that gives skin its colour. Although all people have roughly the same number of melanocytes, the amount of melanin produced varies between individuals. More melanin is produced by dark-skinned people, but repeated exposure to sunlight stimulates the production of melanin, which is why people get suntanned or freckled. The epidermis also contains **Langerhans cells**, which help protect the body against infection.

Below the epidermis is the thicker layer, called the **dermis**, made up of blood vessels, nerve endings and connective tissue. The dermis nourishes the epidermis. There are two types of fibres in the dermis: the strong and inflexible **collagen** and the flexible **elastin**. Their combined function is to allow flexibility of the skin on movement and returning the skin to its original shape on becoming still.

The dermis also contains the **sebaceous glands**. These glands, which surround and empty into hair follicles and pores, produce the oil **sebum** that lubricates the skin and hair. In addition, nerve endings, hair follicles and sweat glands are found within the dermis.

People may make judgements about others on the basis of their skin appearance. Therefore, skin conditions and diseases can have a profound effect on how people feel psychologically in terms of their confidence and self-esteem (Ersser *et al.*, 2007a). Most non-complex skin conditions can be treated effectively using topical preparations as the first intervention.

THE INFLUENCE OF LIFESPAN ON THE SKIN AND SKIN CARE

Infancy (0–23 months)

The skin takes from six months to a year to be effective as a protective barrier (Ersser *et al.*, 2007b). Skin of newborns should be washed with plain water only until the age of about 1 month. The Department of Health (2007) recommends bathing using a mild cleanser 2–3 times weekly with plain water being used in between these times; otherwise, there is an increased risk of the baby developing sensitive skin (Trotter, 2006). Until the age of 2 years, the child's skin is at risk of dryness and so caution using perfumed products is recommended. Babies and toddlers in nappies risk localised dermatitis (nappy rash), unless nappies are changed frequently and effective hygiene measures are used. If nappy rash is not associated with fungal infection, a plain barrier cream will be effective. Otherwise, an antifungal cream may be prescribed (Gupta & Skinner, 2004). For severe cases, a mild steroid cream may be prescribed for very short-term use (Scheinfeld, 2005). Barrier cream can still be applied after the steroid (British National Formulary, 2009).

Childhood (2–12 years)

Many children will suffer some type of skin infection throughout childhood; close proximity to other children and/or adults through school, play and at home increase the likelihood of the spread of skin infections (Sladden & Johnston, 2005).

Chronic skin conditions such as atopic eczema may develop in early childhood, as young as 6 months. According to the National Institute for Health and Clinical Excellence (NICE; 2007), a child who develops eczema will often also develop allergies and asthma. The severity of the condition may vary but shampoo and bubble baths have been identified as potential triggers for the flare-ups. Many incidences of childhood eczema clear or improve significantly towards adulthood.

Adolescence (13–19 years)

Most adolescents will experience acne (teenage spots) at some point in their adolescence, although individuals vary. Because adolescence also brings social unease and a desire to fit in, acne can cause a decrease in self-esteem and an increase in self-consciousness. It is important therefore that the presence of acne is not dismissed by parents or healthcare professionals. Acne is caused by a natural interaction between increased hormone levels, bacteria in the hair follicle and the sebaceous glands (Thiboutot, 2000). Unfortunately, products to reduce the severity of acne tend to take weeks to show any positive effect and it is vital that teenagers are supported and encouraged to complete the course of treatment(s). According to NICE (2001), prolonged or severe acne that risks causing psychological trauma or permanent scarring should be referred for specialist assessment/treatment. Otherwise, the severity and frequency of acne will usually lessen towards adulthood for around 95% of teenagers (Ravenscroft, 2005).

Adulthood (20–64 years)

Many childhood skin conditions will either be reduced in severity or the maturing adult will have found coping mechanisms and be more inclined to follow skin care regimes.

Pregnancy can increase oil production from the sebaceous glands, causing a recurrence of acne, particularly if the condition was troublesome previously. The skin becomes more sensitive than usual and its colour may change, especially over the face. Melasma, as this is known, causes dark, uneven spots to appear most commonly on the forehead and cheeks. This is due to increased pigmentation caused by a change in hormone levels and is reversed after the pregnancy ends.

Many of the changes associated with ageing begin for women around the time of the menopause. However, these same changes can be noted in males too.

Older age (65+ years)

The structure of the skin changes as a normal part of the ageing process. Skin cells may not be replaced as quickly as they are shed. This leads to skin which is thinner and friable (easily torn) (Pringle & Penzer, 2002). Collagen loses its elasticity so that skin becomes looser, wrinkled and skin folds can develop. Older skin is more prone to trauma and pressure damage. Healing times are increased after any skin trauma due to reduced circulation (Burr & Penzer, 2005) and the slowed production of new skin cells. The changes associated with ageing can also affect the skin's ability to act as a barrier to infection. The epidermis thins and corneocytes (skin cells) do not stick together as effectively, which reduces their ability to bind water. This causes drying of the skin (Lawton, 2007). The immaturity of anatomical structures in very pre-term babies causes dry skin for the same reason.

THE INFLUENCE OF THE DEPENDENCE–INDEPENDENCE CONTINUUM ON SKIN HEALTH AND SKIN CARE

The ability to manage skin problems independently is influenced not only by physical and cognitive ability but also by the severity of the skin problem, the site(s) of the condition and the patient's knowledge both about the condition(s) and the treatments. Patients need information about how to maintain healthy skin, what can cause skin problems (e.g. detergents, allergies or sun burn) and how to manage any skin condition in order to regain skin health or prevent deterioration. Patients may not be aware of what topical treatments will be helpful or have knowledge of how to use them effectively.

Skin health can be adversely affected by poor physical health in terms of illness or injury, including dehydration, pressure, trauma, vitamin deficiency and post-surgical procedures. Poor mental health can impact either on skin conditions, which become worse under stress, or on a person's motivation and ability to maintain their own skin health. Social and environmental influences that can cause poor skin health include what a person does for employment or leisure.

ASSESSMENT AND TREATMENT OF COMMON SKIN CONDITIONS

Dry skin (xerosis)

Dry skin can occur for a variety of reasons (Box 8.2). Many people will experience episodes of dry skin at some time, which for most may only present as a minor, infrequent and short-lived irritant. However, for others, dry skin can become a chronic condition that increases the risk of infections and further skin disorders, such as psoriasis and eczema (Voegeli, 2007).

Dry skin may also be a symptom of a separate condition or disease process such as digestive disorders, thyroid imbalance or renal failure.

If the skin lacks natural moisture or the skin is unable to retain moisture, a cycle of poor desquamation and increasingly dry skin is started. Once this cycle begins, the risk of developing secondary conditions such as flaking, inflammation, dermatitis and infection is increased. Therefore, the healthcare professional must be vigilant for skin changes and, particularly in the case of older people, not attribute dry skin to the normal ageing process.

Box 8.2 Common causes of dry skin

- Any decline in production of the protein filaggrin (found in the epidermis) causes skin dryness, including excessive peeling of dry skin.
- Continuous use of soap on the skin can increase the pH to 7.5 from a normal 5.5; the chemical changes and reaction to perfumes can leave the skin feeling dry and taut.
- Any illness which causes a reduction in fluid intake or a prolonged temperature (pyrexia) can result in dry, dehydrated skin.
- Bathing daily (particularly older people) without replacing natural skin emollients.
- Low humidity environments, e.g. hospitals with dry warm air can make dry skin conditions worse.
- Zinc deficiency.
- Some treatments and medications such as radiotherapy and diuretics have dry skin as a known side effect.
- People with dark skin have naturally dryer skin, which is more susceptible to all of the above factors.

(*Source:* Norman, 2003; Burr & Penzer, 2005; Lawton, 2007)

Common symptoms of dry skin

- Dull appearance.
- Rough and uneven to the touch.
- Cracks in the skin.
- Fissures (a cleft or groove).
- Skin may appear scaly or flaky with patchy discoloured areas.
- Oedema (swelling) may be obvious in the surrounding skin, indicating infection.
- The patient may report tightness of the affected area.
- Itching (pruritis), tingling or even pain may be present.

(Norman, 2003; Voegeli, 2007)

Management of dry skin

Emollients (see below) should be used as soap substitutes in order to maintain a normal skin pH. Drying skin thoroughly in order to prevent maceration and further skin drying is important. Skin should be patted dry and not briskly rubbed, to prevent weakening, trauma or abrasions. Moisturising or barrier cream should be smoothed into the skin at least twice daily or according to prescription (any topical treatment should not be rubbed into the skin but smoothed on gently to avoid skin irritation).

When applying topical treatments, the direction of the hair growth should be followed, as rubbing against the hair growth can cause pain, irritation and even infection of the hair follicles (British National Formulary, 2009).

Contact dermatitis

Skin inflammation is caused by direct contact with a substance; contact dermatitis is a term for a skin reaction resulting from exposure to allergens (allergic contact dermatitis) or irritants (irritant contact dermatitis) (Bourke *et al.*, 2001). Many things in everyday life can provoke contact dermatitis, for example latex, nickel (some watches and earrings), detergents, cosmetics, plants and others. Contact dermatitis occurs when the body comes into contact with a substance which it deems foreign; the resulting inflammation is the immune response to the substance (Belsito, 2005) (Figure 8.2).

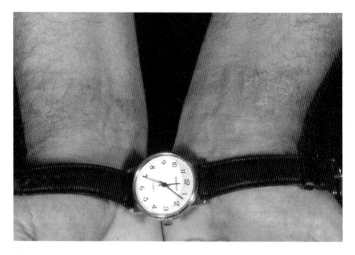

Figure 8.2 Contact dermatitis. From Buxton PK, Morris-Jones R (2009) *ABC of Dermatology*, 5th edn. Reproduced with permission from Wiley-Blackwell.

Dermatitis can be subdivided into different types characterised by slightly different presentations of symptoms or caused by different reactions (Table 8.1). Patch testing can be carried out to identify the causes and irritants which exacerbate the condition (Mark & Slavin, 2006).

Symptoms (acute)

- Itch: generalised or local to area of contact.
- Erythema (redness of the skin due to increased blood supply).
- Presence of papules (small raised areas clustered together on the skin).
- Skin may blister.
- Skin may be wet/weeping.
- Symptoms (chronic).
- Dryness.
- Fissures and cracks in the skin.
- Lichenification (thickening of the skin).

(Belsito, 2005)

Table 8.1 Types of contact dermatitis and their causes

Type of dermatitis	Cause
Atopic	a hereditary tendency to experience immediate allergic reactions because of the presence of an antibody in the skin
Acute irritant	exposure to strong or caustic irritants causing an acute reaction at the site of contact
Chronic irritant	repetitive exposure to weaker, 'wet', irritants, e.g. detergents or 'dry' irritants, such as dust. Can affect a wider area of skin
Subjective irritant	a change in sensation on the skin soon after contact but without evidence of skin changes usually after application of a preparation to the skin, e.g. cosmetics
Allergic reaction	the immune system becomes sensitised to one or more allergens, causing a reaction in the skin
Phototoxic	occurs when the allergen or irritant is activated by sunlight

(*Source:* Bourke *et al.*, 2001; Smith, 2004)

Management of dermatitis

Patients will require education and encouragement to recognise and avoid (if possible) situations where they may be subject to exposure to the irritants. However, avoiding all irritants may not be possible, particularly if contact with irritants are part of a person's occupation (e.g. hairdressing or bricklaying). Protective equipment will be required in these cases (e.g. gloves) to avoid contact with irritants and the use of barrier creams and emollients to minimise the effects of irritants should be advised (Saary *et al.*, 2005). Severe cases of dermatitis may require topical preparations (e.g. corticosteroids) and protective bandaging of the affected sites in conjunction with topical applications. The use of ordinary crêpe bandages or crêpe/cotton mix bandages are effective for protection and tubular bandages may also be used, such as Tubigauze and Stockinette, for large affected areas of the body such as the trunk or legs.

Psoriasis

Psoriasis is a chronic skin condition, in which skin cells reproduce too quickly. Plaque psoriasis is the most common type and affects

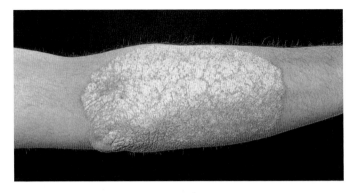

Figure 8.3 Psoriasis. From Graham-Brown R, Burns T (2007) *Lecture Notes: Dermatology.* Reproduced with permission from Wiley-Blackwell.

approximately 2% of people in the UK (Camisa, 2004). The life-cycle of skin cells is more rapid than usual and as a result new cells are produced before old cells die and shed from the skin. This results in a build-up of cells on the skin, which appear as dry, crusty and/or flaky patches (plaques) on areas of the skin. These affected areas are covered with silvery scales, which shed easily (Figure 8.3) (Penzer, 2008).

The condition, which can cause intense itching and a burning sensation, can be unpredictable and fluctuate in severity often becoming worse for no apparent reason. Although psoriasis can affect any areas of the body, the most common areas include:

- Elbows.
- Knees.
- Lower back.

Less common areas include:

- Nails: causes discoloration and abnormal growth.
- Scalp: causes extreme itching and occasional temporary hair loss.
- Folds and creases in the skin: the groin, armpits and under the breast present as smooth red patches.

The exact cause is unknown, but there is a known connection to a lowered immune system in which diseases of the immune system can cause exacerbation of the condition. There may also be familial links towards a tendency to develop the condition (Camisa, 2004). Triggers include stress, injury to the skin, smoking and alcohol use plus the use of certain medications such as anti-inflammatory drugs and beta-blockers (British National Formulary, 2009).

Treatment
Treatments fall into three categories:

- Oral and injected medication: drugs which decrease the production of skin cells are used for moderate psoriasis, whereas drugs which affect the immune response tend to be reserved for the severest cases of psoriasis.
- Phototherapy: the skin is carefully exposed to certain types of light, either natural or ultraviolet A or B. The treatment tends to be more successful if combined with topical treatments.
- Topical: prescribed topical medication can be used for varying severity. Emollients may be effective with mild cases. The most common preparations continue to contain coal tar or Vitamin D.

(British National Formulary, 2009)

Patients may stop using the treatment too quickly because no improvement is noticed (Penzer, 2008), so part of assessment should include what patients have tried and for how long. Psoriasis has a psychological and emotional impact and this is an important part of the assessment process. Feelings of low self-esteem and anxiety in particular are common amongst people living with this condition. This can be made worse at times by ignorance in the general population around the appearance and perceived infection risk from the person with the condition.

Eczema
Eczema causes the skin to become dry, thickened, itchy and red. People with atopic eczema have reduced lipid barrier of the skin

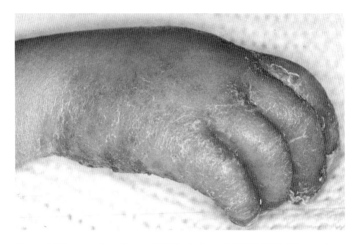

Figure 8.4 Eczema. From Buxton PK, Morris-Jones R (2009) *ABC of Dermatology*, 5th edn. Reproduced with permission from Wiley-Blackwell.

resulting in an increased water loss and dry skin (National Institute for Health and Clinical Excellence, 2007). There are similarities between eczema (Figure 8.4) and psoriasis in that there are familial an immune links to the presence of the condition. Children are commonly affected and the condition will reduce in severity or disappear by adulthood in around two-thirds of cases.

Causes, however, differ in that allergies (e.g. to cows' milk and certain foods plus exposure to animals and dust) can trigger the condition. The majority of childhood eczema presents before the age of 1 year (National Institute for Health and Clinical Excellence, 2007). Ten to fifteen per cent of children have the condition to some degree; this figure reduces to around 5% of adults (Holden & Parrish, 1998).

Poorly managed eczema causes, at times, uncontrollable itching, which in turn can tear the skin. The patient is therefore susceptible to both bacterial and fungal infections (National Institute for Health and Clinical Excellence, 2007).

Like all skin conditions, eczema can cause poor metal health through low self-esteem, or feelings of being bullied or harassed because of the appearance of the skin, and children may become withdrawn and more dependent on their parent(s)/carers (National Institute for Health and Clinical Excellence, 2007).

Treatment

Topical treatment is usually through the use of topical corticosteroids or emollients with antibiotics or antifungals prescribed for any infected phase. Patients should be warned that topical preparations might cause a stinging sensation. Encouraging small children in particular to wear cotton gloves at night can prevent trauma to the skin through scratching during sleep.

Once the acute phase is over, the patient may be prescribed topical preparations less often to prevent the condition flaring up again.

Impetigo

Impetigo is a common, highly contagious bacterial infection of the superficial layers of the skin. Typically associated with poor skin hygiene, it is usually identified as either primary or secondary and bullous or non-bullous (Box 8.3) (George & Rubin, 2003).

Owing to the infectious nature of the condition, impetigo is common in young children and adults who live and/or work in close contact, for example nurseries and care homes (Sladden & Johnston, 2004). Although when untreated impetigo may resolve spontaneously after approximately three weeks, sometimes

---

Box 8.3 Types of impetigo

- Primary impetigo: there is direct bacterial infection of healthy skin.
- Secondary impetigo: infection is a complication of another underlying skin disease (particularly eczema, scabies) or trauma that breaks the skin barrier, e.g. insect bites, burns or IV drug use.
- Bullous impetigo: found usually over the trunk and appearing as rapidly spreading blisters (bullae), which are brownish in colour. This type is more likely to cause the patient to feel unwell.
- Non-bullous impetigo: small pustules that run into each other (most commonly round the nose and mouth) and appear as yellowish-brown crusts.

it can develop into more serious conditions, such as cellulitis, or abscesses may form (Koning *et al.*, 2003).

Treatment

Treatment is usually by topical antibiotic if only a small area of skin is affected. However, if the patient feels systemically unwell or a large area(s) of skin is affected, oral antibiotics may be prescribed (British National Formulary, 2009). Scrupulous personal hygiene and the exclusive use of washing equipment and towels are needed to prevent cross-infection and personal re-infection.

USE OF EMOLLIENTS

Many treatments for conditions that cause dry skin include the use of different types of emollient. Indicated for all dry or scaling disorders (British National Formulary, 2009), emollients can help the skin to repair, plus they soothe, smooth and hydrate the skin. Emollients are grease-based which when applied to the skin can either prevent water loss from the skin (occlusive emollients) or can draw skin from the dermis to the epidermis (Ersser *et al.*, 2007a). During washing, emollients can be added for use as a soap substitute; this maintains the normal pH of the skin and prevents drying of the skin. After washing, emollients can be applied directly to the skin either as a lotion, cream or as an ointment (Table 8.2) in order to moisturise the skin and to prevent water loss.

Emollients can also be combined with other preparations to reduce the itch in skin, to increase exfoliation and can improve the barrier effect of the skin (Ersser *et al.*, 2007a, 2007b).

Side effects of emollient use are infrequent but include (British National Formulary, 2009):

- Contact dermatitis.
- Folliculitis (inflammation of the hair follicles).
- Increased temperature (interference with the body's natural ability to sweat and cool down).
- Increased risk of slipping in the bath or shower.

Table 8.2 Emollient types and descriptions

Emollient types	Definition
Bath additives	Added to water (bath or basin) and are not rinsed off
Soap substitutes	Have cleansing properties and are rinsed off the skin
Lotions	Topical application:
	Contain the least amount of grease and oil and are the lightest and most easily absorbed of the emollients
Creams	Topical application:
	Higher oil content than lotion which is absorbed by the skin
Ointments	Topical application:
	High grease and oil content. Is the most obvious when applied, tends to sit on top of the skin longer before absorption and can stain clothing
	Ointments are effective for very dry skin

(*Source:* Burr & Penzer, 2005; Cooper *et al.*, 2005)

Occasionally, emollient creams may nip when first applied to very dry skin. This normally settles after a few days of treatment but may be a reaction to a preservative in the cream and a medical referral may be needed.

One of the common problems with using emollients is determining how much to use per application. Prescriptions for topic preparations are often vague but the current guidance from the British National Formulary (2009) provides general adult guidelines for a weekly amount based on twice-daily applications (Table 8.3). The equivalent amounts are not appropriate for corticosteroid use.

Procedure: Application of topical emollient
Equipment

- Medication prescription sheet.
- Topical preparation(s) as required.
- Personal protective equipment (PPE) (gloves, if required, and apron).

Table 8.3 Topical preparation dose

Weekly amount/twice daily use	Creams/Ointments	Lotions
Face	15–30 g	100 ml
Both hands	25–50 g	200 ml
Scalp	50–100 g	200 ml
Both arms or both legs	100–200 g	200 ml
Trunk	400 g	500 ml
Groin and genitals	15–25 g	100 ml

(*Source:* British National Formulary, 2009)

NB: Use a clean technique for this procedure.

Action	Rationale
Explain each step of any procedure or examination to the patient and gain their consent	Ensures the patient understands the process and encourages their cooperation
Ensure that the patient is washed or socially clean before applying the preparation	
If washed, skin should be patted dry but left slightly moist before applying leave-on emollient	Moisture is trapped by the preparation, increasing effectiveness and decreasing the number of applications required
Check the prescription and follow local medicine administration guidelines before applying the preparation	Nursing & Midwifery Council's (2008) standards must be adhered to
Ensuring privacy, assist the patient into a comfortable position and remove clothing if/as required	
Check before administration that there are no new concerns about the patient's skin	
Check the expiry date of the preparation	Ensures the preparation is safe to administer
Decontaminate hands	Minimises the risk of cross-infection
Wear gloves if desired/indicated	Gloves are not necessary but may be worn according to clinical judgement or local guidelines

Action	Rationale
Using a pump dispenser or measuring spoon, extract the required amount (or measured portion) of emollient as per prescription	Emollients (particularly creams) are prone to contamination if hands are used to extract the preparation. Pump dispensers and spoons are more accurate in measuring prescribed doses
Smooth the emollient gently over the skin in the direction of hair growth. Do not rub in	Rubbing vigorously can irritate the skin. Going against the direction of hair growth can result in folliculitis (inflammation) if the hair follicle is irritated
Repeat the procedure using measured doses until the area(s) of skin have been treated as prescribed	
Allow the emollient preparation to be absorbed for at least 30 minutes before applying any other topical preparation	Applying other products to moisturised skin may either increase or decrease the potency
Assist the patient to dress if required and return them to a comfortable position with access to the nurse call system	
Remove and dispose of equipment, including PPE, according to local policy	
Decontaminate hands	Prevents cross-infection
Record the nursing intervention and evaluation in the appropriate patient documents. Identify any requirement for reassessment	Ensures continuity of care

(*Source:* Burr & Penzer, 2005, Ersser *et al.*, 2007a; Watkins 2008)

Points to note with emollient therapy

- This procedure may need to be repeated every 2–4 hours, depending on the severity of the patient's condition.
- Intensive use of emollients will reduce the need for steroid therapy; the ratio of use should be 10|:|1 emollient to steroids.
- Emollient therapy should be applied liberally and the patient educated as to the benefits of emollient therapy.

- When discussing emollients with patients, nurses should always refer to complete emollient therapy, which includes the use of bath oils, soap substitutes and moisturisers.

There is little clinical evidence to choose between many of the preparations available and so patient choice and preference are important both for perceived effectiveness and compliance with the therapy (Voegeli, 2007; Watkins, 2008).

Hygiene of the skin is an important factor in treating and improving common skin conditions. Any method of washing which the patient chooses or requires should not be undertaken until the prescribed care and type of topical preparation required is assessed. All registered and non-registered nurses must ensure that the Nursing & Midwifery Council's (2008) standards are adhered to.

BED MAKING

Once the patient is washed, has had all hygiene needs attended to and topical applications applied, the bedding will require attention. Bedding (i.e. sheets, blankets, pillow cases etc.) accumulate high levels of bacteria from skin, infected wound sites and faecal flora. Careless bed making carries the risk of organisms being spread throughout the environment either on the hands of healthcare workers or through the air. Practices such as using chairs or commodes as hangers for linen, dropping linen on the floor and carrying linen through the clinical environment contribute to the spread of infection (Horton & Parker, 2002).

There is debate about whether clean linen on a daily basis is ritualistic practice. It may not be necessary to change bedding every day for all patients and the decision should be made using clinical judgement. Patient comfort must be a consideration, as should the risk of the build-up of bacteria from the patient or external sources.

The bed can be made with the patient out of bed sitting in a chair if the patient is well enough. However, ill patients or those with mobility problems may need to stay in bed for the procedure.

Changing the bedding enhances patient comfort and the nurse can take the opportunity to position the patient in bed in a way that best suits their needs. During the procedure, as with bed bathing, the condition of the patient can be observed, including skin state. The safety and function of equipment being used can also be checked. This is particularly relevant with the technology relating to beds as new and sophisticated beds are becoming increasingly common in clinical areas.

Bed types and equipment
Profiling beds
These electrically adjustable beds can be used to change the patient's position according to their needs (profile). They are manufactured in three or four sections, which can move independently of the others. The top of the bed can be raised to allow the patient to eat or drink more comfortably or to relieve breathlessness. The knee area can be raised to prevent slipping down the bed, reducing the risk of shearing type pressure sores. The risk of injury to the nurse is reduced, as there is less associated moving and handling. The majority of these beds are also height-adjusting, which reduces back strain. Mattresses that are compatible with the beds should be available and used.

Low beds
These beds are capable of being lowered to within inches of the floor to prevent injury to patients who are at risk of falling from the bed. They are compatible with moving and handling hoists. Care must be taken to use a bed that has a safeguard against patients being trapped under the bed should they fall.

Lateral tilting systems (kinetic beds)
These are mains-powered beds that will turn the person from side to side, thus eliminating the need for turning manually, for example where turning needs to continue throughout the night. They provide pressure relief and assist postural drainage (i.e. drainage of fluid from the lungs). Lateral tilting positioning

systems are designed to be used with traditional hospital beds and some profiling beds.

A longitudinally sectioned mattress is alternately inflated and deflated, which has the effect of tilting the person from side to side.

These units can be controlled by the patient or the carer using a handset or can be set to automatically turn at pre-programmed intervals. It is advisable to use most of these units with bed rails, as they do not have built-in side protection.

They reduce the potential discomfort for patients when being moved and reduce the strain on nurses' backs.

Traditional hospital beds or divan beds in care homes or the patient's own home may not provide adequate protection against the development of pressure sores in certain circumstances (e.g. acute illness, physical frailty, poor nutrition). The use of a pressure-reducing system will have to be considered; the type chosen may impact on how the linen should be arranged to ensure maximum effectiveness.

Mattress types
Pressure-reducing/relieving mattresses
Low-maintenance systems comprise a material that conforms to the shape of the body and redistributes the body weight of a patient over a larger area and therefore reduces the pressure exerted by the body. They include (National Institute for Health and Clinical Excellence, 2003):

- High-specification foam mattresses.
- Convoluted foam mattresses.
- Cubed foam mattresses.
- Gel/fluid/fibre/air-filled mattresses/overlays.

High-tech devices

- Alternating-pressure mattresses/overlays where air-filled sacs or sections inflate and deflate in cycles over different parts of the mattress which then relieve the pressure under the patient.

- Air-fluidised mattresses integral to a bed which electrically circulates warm air through fine ceramic beads and distributes pressure over a larger area.
- Low-air-loss mattresses/overlays/beds where air-filled sacs are kept at a constant pressure.
- Turning beds/frames which can turn the patient through a range of different positions electronically.

(National Institute for Health and Clinical Excellence, 2003)

The bed type must be assessed in order to use the correct bed making technique and materials. Some bed devices may have their performance reduced by making a bed traditionally (e.g. low-air-loss beds and mattresses). Pressure relief is provided when the supporting surface is deep and soft enough to allow the user to partially sink into its surface. These mattresses allow pressure to be evenly distributed along the supporting surface and reduce the accumulation of heat and moisture. The beds can be profiled to alter the position of a user.

These beds and mattresses are for people who have high-dependency needs and who may already have a vulnerable skin condition. They can be used with or without a cover or sheet. Rubber-backed sheets and plastic draw sheets should not be used as they prevent airflow. There are many different types of equipment such as special mattresses which may mean that the bed needs to be made differently from the traditional King's Fund bed. The manufacturer's instructions must be followed to ensure the patient's safety. Always check before making a bed if there is uncertainty about the equipment on or around the bed. There are many different types of beds and bedding which a nurse could encounter (e.g. in care homes or in the patient's own home). An assessment must be made from a moving and handling perspective.

There are certain principles associated with bed making which should be considered and adhered to in order to provide safe patient care and minimise the risk of injury to the nurse. The principles for bed making remain the same whatever the bed, with patient safety, control of infection and moving and handling safety at the centre of decision-making.

Personal safety

Nurses may have to kneel to make some low beds in the patient's own home or some care homes. The risk of infection from the floor should be taken account of and protection from the floor and for the knees is vital. What must be remembered is that the load when making a bed is horizontal rather than the vertical lifts demonstrated in moving and handling. The strain will therefore be on the nurse's arms and shoulders, which are often weaker than the legs (Nelson *et al.*, 2003a). The nurse must consider personal safety, and patient lifts, glide sheets and other moving and handing equipment must be provided in every care setting.

Where possible, two people should make a bed. This is safer and reduces the need to overstretch. The nurse should always work at one end of the mattress and then the other to avoid overstretching. The nurse should walk up the side of the bed while tucking in bed linen, again to avoid twisting and back strains.

Where possible and safe for the patient have them sit in a chair during bed making. If making a bed with the patient in it, reassure the patient about their safety during the procedure. Some patients may be afraid that they will fall from the bed when asked to roll. Do not use bed rails to balance the patient at the side of the bed – the patient's limbs may slip though the slats, with the possibility of trauma.

Always have the bed at the correct height: too high and the nurse may strain their back reaching over; too low puts an unnecessary strain on the back while bending.

Infection control

Bedclothes should be folded during removal and not shaken – this reduces potential cross-infection.

NEVER put soiled linen on the floor – always place immediately in a receptacle for soiled linen. Ensure the receptacle is not over full, to prevent cross-infection. Place the receptacle for soiled linen next to the bed during the procedure. Wear an apron for bed making and NEVER carry soiled linen through a ward, as there is a risk of cross-infection to patients from infected uniforms. Gloves are not required for general bed making; if there is a high infection risk from removing soiled sheets, gloves may be required. The purpose of the procedure must be assessed and infection control principles applied. For example, if bed making is part of a discharge procedure, full decontamination will be required. The patient may be incontinent or have an infection, the patient may be post-surgery and the bed may be contaminated with blood and decontamination of the mattress will also be required.

Comfort

The patient may become cold so windows should be closed during the procedure. Although sheets should be wrinkle-free, avoid having the bottom sheet tucked in too tight as this may contribute to pressure sores.

Dignity and privacy

Engage the patient in conversation. This is part of their care and assists with the ongoing assessment process. Privacy is vital during bed making and patients may feel vulnerable and exposed during bed making. Ensure that night clothes cover the patient, and avoid prolonged periods where the patient is uncovered.

Provide support and assistance for your patient and always explain what you need them to do and why.

Procedure: Making an unoccupied bed

Equipment

- Trolley with clean linen.
- Carrier or receptacle for used/soiled linen.
- Bed stripper (if not part of the bed).
- PPE.
- Materials for mattress decontamination (according to local policy for infection control).

Action	Rationale
Explain each step of any procedure or examination to the patient and gain their consent	Ensures the patient understands the process and encourages their cooperation
Ensure privacy	Contributes to dignity
Decontaminate hands and put on PPE (gloves are not necessary unless the sheets are contaminated with body fluids)	Reduces cross-infection
Raise the bed height to suit your working height and that of your partner (bed should be raised to suit the shorter partner)	Reduces the risk of back injury
Pull or position the bed stripper from the bottom of the bed end or position two chairs at the bottom of the bed (if no mobile bed stripper is available)	Reduces the risk of dropping soiled linen on the floor
Ensure any equipment is handled with care and according to protocol/ manufacturer's instructions (e.g. integral bed rails, removable bed rails, electrical equipment for profiling beds)	Reduces the risk of accidental trauma/misuse
Position the linen receptacle next to the bed	Reduces the risk of dropping linen accidentally or nurses carrying soiled linen through the clinical area next to their uniforms
Remove the pillows and place soiled pillow cases in the linen receptacle. Place pillows on the bed stripper	The additional weight of pillows can make the bottom sheet difficult to move safely
Loosen the top and bottom bedclothes all around the bed from top to bottom of bed	Allows easier removal of the bed covers
Fold all linen individually. Fold from top to 1/3 way down, repeat to 2/3, fold again and lay each cover on the bed stripper or place directly into used-linen receptacle	Bedclothes are not disturbed; avoids the shaking of the covers. Allows covers to be replaced with ease and minimal disturbance

Action	Rationale
Inspect the mattress for damage or staining	Reduces the risk of cross-infection. All covers should be made of two-way stretch material, to reduce the risk of adding to the shearing forces on a patient's sacral area, in particular – damage to the cover will reduce the effectiveness
Decontaminate the mattress as required according to local infection control policy	Prevents contamination of the new linen from the mattress
Test the bed for bottoming out by spreading the hands and pushing down on the middle third of the mattress. The base of the bed should not be felt through the mattress	Checks that the mattress is still of a suitable standard for patient care. Mattresses if not cared for may only last up to 18 months in a hospital environment
Turn the mattress according to manufacturer's guidelines (some mattresses have numbers in each corner to guide the turning phases)	Systematic turning of the mattress (i.e. flipping and rotating end to end) prolongs its life by spreading the load from the patient
Unfold a clean sheet lengthways with the wide hem at the top of the bed. Ensure that the central fold (the 'V' shape) faces upwards	Linen has a rough and a smooth side according to the weave. Traditionally, the laundry service will fold sheets with the smooth side upwards. Ensuring the smooth side is next to the patient's skin increases comfort
Ensuring that the sheet is evenly positioned over the mattress, tuck the sheet under the mattress using mitred corners (see below)	Prevents slippage of the sheets during or after the process
Assess the purpose of the bed making (e.g. admission bed, post-surgical bed or making a bed for a current patient). Follow local policy for each circumstance	

Continued

Action	Rationale
For a current patient: place a clean sheet over the bottom sheet allowing enough material at the top to fold over the blankets. Ensure that the centre fold (the 'V' shape) faces downwards towards the patient	
Before tucking the sheet in loosely at the sides, fold the sheet into a pleat at the bottom and tuck in loosely using mitred corners	Allows the patient to move their feet but prevents feet from becoming cold owing to the bedclothes have moved away from the foot of the bed
Replace the blanket(s) one by one. Each blanket should be folded slightly into a pleat at the bottom of the bed before tucking in loosely using mitred corners	The patient must have enough room to move freely in the bed. Tightly tucking in linen can increase the risk of pressure sores through restricted movement and can cause panic in people with cognitive difficulties. Not tucking in linen can cause a restless patient to become cold if the covers shift. Covers not tucked in risk partially slipping onto the floor, increasing the risk of cross-infection and tripping accidents
Replace clean pillow cases and place pillows on the bed	
Fold the top covers and sheets neatly. Enough linen should be folded over to allow the patient to pull them up and cover their shoulders while sleeping	Prevents the patient from becoming cold
Ensure that all brakes are applied	Reduces the risk of accidents
Ensure all equipment in use is back in place and in working order	Reduces the risk of malfunctioning equipment and/or trauma to the patient

Action	Rationale
Ensure that the bed is lowered to a height suitable for your patient's requirements	Reduces trauma risk if the patient climbs or falls out of bed
Replace bed rails if it has been assessed that they are required	As above, patient may require the bed rails to assist with independent mobility
Clean the patient's locker, bed table and any other equipment following local infection control policy	
Remove the used-linen receptacle to the appropriate area in the ward	Reduces cross-infection
Do not leave the receptacle over full: tie up the receptacle according to local policy and replace with an empty one	Reduces cross-infection
Remove and dispose of PPE decontaminate your hands	Reduces cross-infection
Report any deficits or concerns to the ward manager, completing any paperwork as required	Ensures the safe maintenance of equipment

Procedure: Making an occupied bed
Equipment

- Trolley with clean linen.
- Carrier or receptacle for used/soiled linen.
- Bed stripper (if not part of the bed).
- PPE.

If required:

- Fresh night clothes for the patient.
- Absorbent continence aids.

NB: Ideally, two nurses should carry out this procedure.

Action	Rationale
Explain each step of any procedure or examination to the patient and gain their consent	Ensures the patient understands the process and encourages their cooperation
Ensure privacy	Contributes to dignity
Decontaminate hands and put on PPE (gloves are not necessary unless the sheets are contaminated with body fluids)	Reduces cross-infection
Raise the bed height to suit your working height and that of your partner (bed should be raised to suit the shorter partner)	Reduces the risk of back injury
Pull bed stripper from the bottom of the bed end or position two chairs at the bottom of the bed	Reduces the risk of dropping soiled linen on the floor
Ensure any equipment is handled with care and according to protocol/ manufacturer's instructions (e.g. IV infusions, drains, urinary catheters etc.)	Reduces the risk of accidental trauma/misuse
Position the linen receptacle next to the bed	Reduces the risk of dropping linen accidentally or nurses carrying soiled linen through the clinical area next to their uniforms
Loosen the top and bottom bedclothes all round the bed from top to bottom of bed	Allows easier removal of the bed covers
Remove as many pillows as the patient can tolerate or is safe	The additional weight of pillows can make the bottom sheet difficult to move safely
Fold the top bed covers individually. Fold from top to 1/3 way down, repeat to 2/3, fold again and lay each cover on the bed stripper or place directly into used-linen receptacle	Bedclothes are not disturbed; avoids the shaking of the covers. Allows covers to be replaced with ease and minimal disturbance
Strip the top cover(s) as far as the blanket next to the patient	Avoids exposing the patient
Slip out the sheet next to the patient from under the blanket and place directly into the used/soiled-linen receptacle	Maintains the patient's dignity
Using appropriate manual handling techniques and equipment, roll your patient to one side of the bed with one nurse supporting them safely	Avoids the risk of injury to the nurse or patient
If possible (and required), remove any absorbent continence aids	Reduces the disturbance to the patient through additional rolling

Action	Rationale
Roll the bottom sheet evenly towards the patient's back, exposing approximately 1/2–2/3 of the mattress	
Decontaminate the mattress of bodily fluids if required according to local infection control policy	Prevents contamination of the new linen from the mattress
Unfold a clean sheet lengthways with the wide hem at the top of the bed. Ensure that the central fold (the 'V' shape) faces upwards	Linen has a rough and a smooth side according to the weave. Traditionally, the laundry service will fold sheets with the smooth side upwards. Ensuring the smooth side is next to the patient's skin increases comfort
Leaving 1/4 of the sheet over the edge of the bed, roll the remainder towards the patient ensuring that the clean and used sheets do not come into contact	Prevents contamination of the new linen from soiled linen
Tuck the sheet under the mattress using mitred corners (see below)	Prevents slippage of the sheets during or after the process
Supporting your patient and using appropriate manual handling techniques and equipment, help the patient to roll over the sheets (an absorbent continence pad can be rolled and placed with the sheets at this stage)	
The nurse at the receiving side then removes the used sheet first, placing it directly into the used-linen receptacle and decontaminates the bed if required	
The clean sheet is then rolled out smoothly and tucked in at the other side of the bed using mitred corners. The sheet should be firmly anchored but not taut	Too tight and unnecessary pressure is put onto the skin
Ensuring that there are no creases in the bottom sheet, return your patient to the bed centre	The bed centre is safest and allows a choice of patient positioning
Remove pillow cases. Place them directly into the used-linen receptacle and replace with clean ones	
Supporting the patient's head, remove any pillows; replace some or all of the clean pillows under the patient immediately	Reduces the risk of discomfort or neck pain or injury to the patient

Continued

303

Action	Rationale
Remove the blanket covering the patient and immediately place a clean sheet over the patient; allow enough material at the top to fold over the blankets. Ensure that the centre fold (the 'V' shape) faces downwards towards the patient	
Before tucking the sheet in loosely at the sides, fold the sheet into a pleat at the bottom and tuck in loosely using mitred corners	Allows the patient to move their feet but prevents feet from becoming cold owing to the bedclothes being moved away from the foot of the bed
Replace the blanket(s) one by one. Each blanket should be folded slightly into a pleat at the bottom of the bed before tucking in loosely using mitred corners	The patient must have enough room to move freely in the bed. Tightly tucking in linen can increase the risk of pressure sores through restricted movement and can cause panic in people with cognitive difficulties. Not tucking in linen can cause a restless patient to become cold if the covers shift. Covers not tucked in risk partially slipping onto the floor, increasing the risk of cross-infection and tripping accidents
Replace the top cover, using half-mitred corners at the bottom, fold the sheets and blankets over the top cover but ensure that your patient's chest is covered and that they will be warm enough	
Ensure that you have not tucked the linen in too tightly and that the patient can draw the covers as high as is comfortable	Allows patient choice and keeps the patient warm
Ensure that all brakes are applied	Reduces the risk of accidents
Ensure all equipment in use is back in place and in working order	Reduces the risk of malfunctioning equipment and/or trauma to the patient

Action	Rationale
Ensure that the bed is lowered to a height suitable for your patient's requirements	Reduces trauma risk if the patient climbs or falls out of bed
Replace bed rails if it has been assessed that they are required	As above, patient may require the bed rails to assist with independent mobility
Ensure that your patient is comfortable and has access to their locker and the nurse call system	Increases patient dignity and safety
Remove the used-linen receptacle to the appropriate area in the ward	Reduces cross-infection
Do not leave the receptacle over full; tie up the receptacle according to local policy and replace with an empty one	Reduces cross-infection
Remove and dispose of PPE decontaminate your hands	Reduces cross-infection

Mitred (hospital or envelope) corners

Making a bed with mitred corners ensures that the sheets stay anchored and creases are reduced. This improves comfort for the patient and prevents pressure sores developing from the creases.

- Start at the top end of the mattress; tuck the sheet evenly under, pulling it taut and smooth.
- Slide your hand under the side edge of sheet about 30 cm down from the top/bottom of the mattress and draw upwards into a diagonal fold.
- Lay this fold up over the mattress.
- The part of sheet left hanging is tucked under the mattress holding your hands palm down to protect your knuckles from the hard underside of the bed.
- Take the upper fold from over the mattress, let it hang and tuck in under mattress.
- Repeat at the other side and then at the bottom corners.
- The sheet will now be anchored. Linen on top of the patient can be anchored in the same way at the foot of the bed. Debate remains as to whether all top linen should be mitred together or individually. The consideration is the patient: if the

patient is likely to be warm and some linen may be removed, tuck individually to save the remainder of the linen being dislodged.

The bed – if a profiling bed – can then be altered to a position best suited to the patient's needs. Additional pillows will be required to assume positions not possible with profiling beds or for beds which are static.

POSITIONING THE PATIENT COMFORTABLY IN BED

Patients need to be moved in bed for several reasons. Maintaining one particular position causes muscle fatigue. Patients will develop pressure sores if they are not moved. Frequency of position changes will be dictated by the patient's pressure sore risk, the type of mattress used and an evaluation of pressure-relieving interventions.

Complications of bed rest can occur in a relatively short time, particularly for older people (Box 8.4). Although moving patients in bed will not counteract the effects of all physiological/psychological changes, the effects can be reduced.

Patients who must stay in bed much of the time should be kept as comfortable as possible to prevent body deformities. A patient

---

Box 8.4 Potential complications of bed rest in older people

- Pressure sores.
- Postural hypotension (falling blood pressure on sitting or standing).
- Hypercalcaemia.
- Bone resorption.
- Pneumonia.
- Thromboembolism (DVT).
- Urinary incontinence.
- Constipation.
- Depression.
- Anxiety.
- Muscle weakness.
- Contractures.

(*Source:* Kane *et al.*, 2003)

---

with any form of paralysis may not be aware that they have been left in a dangerous position. The patient's body should be aligned straight to prevent injury. Respiration and digestion are improved if the patient is positioned properly and pillows can be used as needed to support the patient's head, neck, arms and hands for comfort. A slanted footboard can support the patient's feet at right angles to the leg (a normal angle) and to prevent foot drop.

Moving and handling technology

Before positioning the patient, the patient's moving and handling assessment must be referred to. Moving and handling equipment identified for use with the patient must be used. By using equipment, the patient's dignity is promoted, as awkward handing situations can prove embarrassing and frightening for a patient (Nelson, 2003b). Assistive patient handling equipment can be selected to match a patient's ability to assist in their own movement, thereby promoting independence. The risk of injury to the patient (e.g. skin tears and pressure sores through friction or shearing) is reduced. The safety of the nurse is enhanced because the equipment, if used properly, is designed to complement the capabilities of the human body (Owen, 2000). Without equipment, when lifting or repositioning a resident in bed, the bed width prevents the caregiver from bending their knees to assume the proper posture for lifting. The forward bending needed to move patients stresses the nurse's spine at its most vulnerable position (Collins *et al.*, 2004).

Most clinical areas have a no-lift policy, which should be explained carefully to the patient. This policy applies to patients in bed too. Glide sheets and slides should be used to move a patient over the bed surface, and should a non-weight-bearing patient require to be raised from the bed, a hoist should be used.

Procedure: Preparing a patient for a change of position

The following actions should be undertaken (and some or all of the following equipment used) as part of any procedure to change a patient's position in bed. This procedure is for patients without spinal complications; specialised moves are outwith the remit of this book.

Possible equipment required for positioning a patient

- Additional pillows.
- Foot board.
- Wedges.
- Moving and handling aids.
- Balance aids.
- PPE (apron and gloves).

Action	Rationale
Refer to the patient's moving and handling assessment to determine which moves are safe for the patient and what equipment is needed	Individualises care and promotes safety
Collect equipment – moving and handling aids/pillows/balance aids	The patient should not be left unaided, for safety reasons
Assess how many nurses are required on the basis of the moving and handling assessment	
Decontaminate hands and put on PPE	
Introduce yourself and explain the procedure to the patient; discuss how they can contribute	
Draw curtains and shut the door	Increases privacy
Check that the brakes are applied on the bed	Reduces the risk of accidental injury
Raise the bed to a comfortable working level	
Remove/lower any bed rails which are in use	
Check for any medical equipment being used with the patient (e.g. urinary catheter, IV infusion, wound drains)	
Fold bedding to the patient's hips but no lower, unless necessary	Promotes privacy and dignity

Action	Rationale
Remove all pillows currently being used to maintain a position. Where possible, leave only one or two pillows under the patient's head	Too many pillows provide a barrier to safe movement and may hurt the nurse
Recheck and remove/make safe any equipment attached to the bed or the patient (e.g. pumps, IV infusions, urinary catheters)	Avoids injury to the patient and protects the equipment
Prepare the patient verbally for the change of position	

Procedure: General roll onto the patient's left side

NB: When re-positioning a patient, the nurse should check the skin and bony protuberances for signs of pressure, be aware of pain on movement and protect the patient from injury.

Action	Rationale
Ensure that there are the correct number of nurses for the procedure	Prevents injury to the patient or nurse(s)
Explain to the patient the procedure about to take place	The patient is less likely to resist the position change and less likely to injure the nurse
Two nurses ideally should be standing at the side the patient will roll to	The patient will feel safer and the nurses' backs are at less risk
If the patient is already lying on one side, assist them back onto their back	
Gently turn the patient's head towards the direction of the roll (e.g. left)	
Flex (bend) the patient's right leg at the knee and sweep the patient's right leg over their left	The patient is prepared for the move and there is an ergonomically easier move
Ensure the patient's left arm is free from under them and crossed over their chest; bring their right arm over the front of their body and cross over their chest too	

Continued

Action	Rationale
With the nurses standing at the patient's shoulders/waist and waist/knees, the patient should be pulled gently towards both nurses with hands on the patient's shoulder and hip	Moves the patient without placing strain on the patient's neck or twisting the patient
The nurse at the back of the patient can then insert any glide sheets, carry out hygiene measures or sort continence aids/clothing	
The patient should not be left in this position, but it is a precursor for placing the patient in a comfortable position	

Supine position (Figure 8.5)

This position is also known as the recumbent position.

Common uses

- For physical examination, e.g. abdominal examination
- Relaxed position, e.g. for sleeping
- Aids blood flow, e.g. to kidneys in older people.
- Part of a turning programme for pressure sore prevention.

Cautions

- Pressure sore risk if the position is maintained too long.
- Restricts chest expansion for breathing; therefore is not suitable for people with breathing difficulties.
- Difficulty carrying out activities of living, e.g. eating and drinking or communicating.

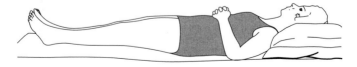

Figure 8.5 Supine/recumbent/horizontal position.

Procedure

- Roll the patient from their side onto their back.
- Align the patient straight in the bed (head, neck, spine, hips knees and feet).
- Place the patient's arms comfortably at their side.
- Place one or two pillows (according to choice and comfort) under the patient's head/neck about two inches below shoulder level.
- Place a footboard at the patient's feet to keep them at right angles to their legs (prevents foot drop); place a trochanter roll (see below) if needed along each hip and thigh (prevents the hip joint from rotating outwards).
- Return the bed to a low position, return bedclothes to a comfortable position and ensure the patient has access to the nurse call system.
- Place the bed table in a low position where the patient can reach items needed.

Semi-supine and dorsal positions (Figure 8.6)

A semi-supine position can be achieved by adding pillows under the patient's head and shoulders. The patient's body should be aligned as described above. This position better suits patients

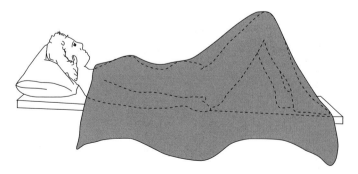

Figure 8.6 Dorsal position.

who have difficulty breathing. Another variation of the supine position is the dorsal position, which is used for vaginal examination/smear testing, perineal cleansing and insertion of an indwelling urinary catheter. The position can make the patient feel very vulnerable and absolute privacy and adequate coverage are essential.

The semi-supine position can be achieved by placing the patient in the supine position; ask the patient to flex their knees and bring their feet up towards their buttocks. The patient should then be asked to place their feet together and relax their knees apart.

Prone position
Lying on the stomach – pillow under head, abdomen and ankles.

Common uses

- Part of turning programme.
- Treatment for burns/sores/spinal injuries.
- Chest drainage (foot of bed raised).

Cautions

- Uncomfortable for any length of time.
- Limits self-movement and care.
- Difficult to eat, drink, talk.

Procedure

- Start with the bed flat and the patient lying on their front with their head turned to one side (left or right), spine straight and legs extended.
- Place their head in the middle of a pillow.
- Place a small pillow under the hips. This relieves pressure on the back and reduces pressure against a female patient's breasts.
- Place a pillow under their arms to reach from the elbow to below the wrists, raising their hands slightly. Their shoulders

and elbows may be flexed or extended, whichever is more comfortable for the patient.

- Place a pillow under their lower legs to prevent pressure on their toes. The patient may be moved down in the bed before starting the procedure, so that their feet extend over the end of the mattress. This allows the foot to assume a normal standing position. However, this may cause the patient to have cold feet and it may not be comfortable.

Lateral position (left and right) (Figure 8.7)
Common uses

- Sleeping.
- Part of turning programme.
- Unconscious patient.
- Lumbar puncture.

Cautions

- Uncomfortable for any length of time.
- Limits self-movement and care.
- Difficult to eat, drink, talk etc.
- Pressure sore risk if maintained too long.

Procedure

- Start with the bed flat and the patient turned on their side. Before positioning the patient on their side, use a glide sheet to move them from their side to the middle of the bed.

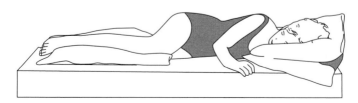

Figure 8.7 Lateral position.

- Place a pillow under their head from under the patient's head down towards the shoulders.
- Position the patient's lower arm so that the shoulder and elbow are flexed and the palm of the hand is facing up.
- Slightly flex the patient's upper arm to rest on the patient's hip or bring it forward and place it on a pillow. The patient's shoulder, elbow and wrist should be at approximately the same height.
- Place a pillow between the patient's legs from above the knee to below the ankle. The patient's hip, knee and ankle should be at approximately the same height.
- The patient's legs may be separated by the pillows and so that the patient is lying around 30° from the mattress or the lower leg can be left straight and the upper leg flexed in front of the patient and supported by the pillow (see above). The patient will be around 45° from the mattress in this position.
- A pillow may be placed behind the patient's back to help maintain the position in the bed.

Sim's position

Sim's position is a variation of the lateral position but the patient only lies on their left side. This position is often used for rectal examination and the administration of suppositories and enemas.

Fowler's position (Figure 8.8)

Fowler's position is sometimes known as the arm chair position.

Common uses

- Aids breathing.
- Post operatively for some surgery, e.g. abdominal.
- Helps eating and drinking.
- Good position to socialise and communicate.

Cautions

- May slide down the bed and cause shearing/friction-related pressure sores.
- Pressure sore risk if maintained too long.

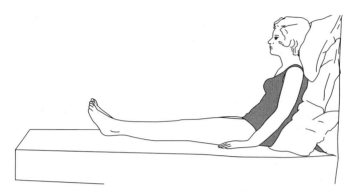

Figure 8.8 Fowler's position.

Procedure

- Move the patient from lying on their back in the middle of the bed towards the top of the bed. (The patient may be able to manage this independently.) Place the patient's bottom at the point where the bed bends (if a profiling bed) or near to the base of the adjustable backrest.
- Raise the head of the bed 30° for a semi-Fowler's position, 45–60° for a normal Fowler's position and 90° for a high Fowler's position.
- The patient may have a pillow at the base of their spine to prevent discomfort from the bed rest (the nurse should be aware that profiling beds can be uncomfortable if the patient is left with too few pillows). Additional pillows should be placed at the back of the patient's shoulders and head.
- Bend the patient's elbows into a comfortable position and place a pillow under each arm to prevent pull on the shoulders and to maintain the patient's balance in the bed.
- Use a footboard or folded pillow to keep feet in position and to prevent the patient from sliding down the bed.

Orthopnoeic position (Figure 8.9)

Common uses

- Drainage of chest wounds.
- Position which is most effective for optimising breathing.
- Patient is more likely to achieve independence in washing etc.
- Prevents further breathing problems.

Cautions

- Not a suitable sleeping position.
- Difficult to maintain.
- Pressure sore risk if maintained too long.

Procedure

- This is a variation of a high Fowler's position at a 90° angle and is used for patients who have difficulty breathing.
- The bedside table is moved across the bed near to the patient's chest and abdomen. Place one or two pillows on top of the table.
- The patient should be able to lean forward across the table comfortably. The patient's arms should be extended to right angles from the body and then raised above the patient's head over or beside the pillows. This position expands the lungs and aids breathing.

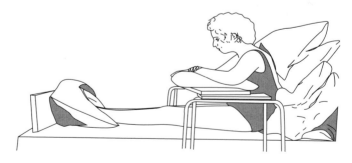

Figure 8.9 Orthopnoeic position.

- The patient should rest their head on the pillows, facing whichever side is comfortable.
- Place another pillow or more low behind the patient's back for support.

CONCLUSION

This chapter has discussed the care of a patient's skin and making their beds, and provides a guide for some of the more common patient positions. Having healthy skin and being comfortable in bed contribute to the patient's well-being. This book has hopefully illustrated the importance of meeting a patient's hygiene needs. The knowledge and nursing interventions are fundamental to quality care. Nurses should be aware that these skills are not just the 'basic care' sometimes spoken of in a derogatory manner in comparison to the more technological and advanced roles that nurses now undertake. Without these skills being carried out for and with patients, the more advanced care will not be as effective as it could be. The fundamentals of care are the aspects of care which patients appreciate when they're carried out well and miss when they're not.

REFERENCES

Belsito DV (2005) Occupational contact dermatitis: Etiology, prevalence, and resultant impairment/disability. *Journal of the American Academy of Dermatology* **53**(2): 303–313.

Bourke J, Coulson I, English J (2001) Guidelines for care of contact dermatitis. *British Journal of Dermatology* **145**(6): 877–885.

British National Formulary (2009) *British National Formulary*, 58th edn. Pharmaceuticals Press, London.

Burr S, Penzer R (2005) Promoting skin health. *Nursing Standard* **19**(36): 57–66.

Camisa C (2004) *Handbook of Psoriasis*, 2nd edn. Blackwell Science, London.

Collins JW, Wolf L, Bell J *et al.* (2004) An evaluation of a 'best practices' musculoskeletal injury prevention program in nursing homes. *Injury Prevention* **10**: 206–211.

Cooper P, Clark M, Bale S (2005) *Best practice statement: Care of the older person's skin.* Wounds UK and 3M Health Care, London.

Department of Health (2007) *Birth to five: 2007 edition.* DH, London.

Ersser SJ, Latter S, Sibley A *et al.* (2007a) Psychological and educational interventions for atopic eczema in children (review). *Cochrane Database of Systematic Reviews*, **3**(CD004054): 1–33. (doi:10.1002/14651858. CD004054.

Ersser SJ, Maguire S, Nicol R *et al.* (2007b) *Best practice for emollient therapy*. Dermatological Nursing, Aberdeen: Dermatology UK.

George A, Rubin G (2003) A systematic review and meta-analysis of treatments for impetigo. *British Journal of General Practice* **53**(491): 480–487.

Gupta AK, Skinner AR (2004) Management of diaper dermatitis. *International Journal of Dermatology* **43**(11): 830–840.

Holden CA, Parish WE (1998) Atopic dermatitis. In: RH Champion, JL Burton, DA Burns *et al.* (eds), *Rook/Wilkinson/Ebling Textbook of Dermatology: Volume 1*, 6th edn. Blackwell Science, Oxford, 681–708.

Horton R, Parker L (2002) *Informed Infection Control Practice*, 2nd edn. Churchill Livingstone, London.

Kane RL, Ouslander JG, Abrass I (2003) *Essentials of Clinical Geriatrics*. McGraw-Hill, New York.

Koning S, Verhagen AP, van Suijlekom-Smit LWA *et al.* (2003) *Interventions for Impetigo (Cochrane Review)*. The Cochrane Library. Issue 2. John Wiley & Sons, Ltd, http://www.thecochranelibrary.com, [accessed 9 March 2009].

Lawton S (2007) Addressing the skin-care needs of the older person. *British Journal of Community Nursing* **12**(5): 203–204, 206, 208.

Mark BJ, Slavin RG (2006) Allergic contact dermatitis. *Medical Clinics of North America* **90**(1): 169–185.

National Institute for Health and Clinical Excellence (2001) *Referral Advice: A guide to appropriate referral from general to specialist services*. NICE, London.

National Institute for Health and Clinical Excellence (2003) *Pressure Ulcer Prevention: Clinical guideline 7*. NICE, London.

National Institute for Health and Clinical Excellence (2007) *Atopic Eczema in Children: Management of atopic eczema in children from birth up to the age of 12 years (NICE guideline)*. NICE, London.

Nelson A, Fragala G, Menzel N (2003a) Myths and facts about back injuries in nursing: Part 1. *American Journal of Nursing* **103**(2): 32–40.

Nelson A, Fragala G, Menzel N (2003b) Safe patient handling and movement. *American Journal of Nursing* **103**(3): 47–52.

Norman RA (2003) Caring for aging skin. *Nursing Homes Long Term Care Management* **52**: 22–24.

Nursing & Midwifery Council (2008) *Standards for Medicines Management*. NMC, London.

Owen BD (2000) Preventing injuries using an ergonomic approach. *AORN Journal* **72**(6): 1031–1036.

Penzer R (2008) Providing patients with information on caring for skin. *Nursing Standard* **23**(9): 49–56.

Pringle F, Penzer R (2002) Normal Skin: Its function and care. In: R Penzer (ed.), *Nursing Care of the Skin*. Butterworth-Heinemann, Oxford, 20–45.

Ravenscroft J (2005) Evidence based update on the management of acne. *Archives of Disease in Childhood Education and Practice Edition* **90**(4): ep98–ep101.

Saary J, Qureshi R, Palda V *et al.* (2005) A systematic review of contact dermatitis treatment and prevention. *Journal of the American Academy of Dermatology* **53**(5): 845–852.

Scheinfeld N (2005) Diaper dermatitis: A review and brief survey of eruptions of the diaper area. *American Journal of Clinical Dermatology* **6**(5): 273–281.

Sladden MJ, Johnston GA (2004) Common skin infections in children. *British Medical Journal* **329**(7457): 95–99.

Sladden MJ, Johnston GA (2005) More common skin infections in children. *British Medical Journal* **330**(7501): 1194–1198.

Smith A (2004) Contact dermatitis: Diagnosis and management. *British Journal of Community Nursing* **9**(9): 365–371.

Thibodeau GA, Patton KT (2008) *Structure & Function of the Body*, 13th edn, Mosby/Elsevier, St Louis.

Thiboutot D (2000) New treatments and therapeutic strategies for acne. *Archives of Family Medicine* **9**(2): 179–187.

Trotter S (2006) Neonatal skincare: Why change is vital. *RCM Midwives Journal* **9**(4): 134–138.

Voegeli D (2007) The role of emollients in the care of patients with dry skin. *Nursing Standard* **22**(7): 62–68.

Watkins P (2008) Using emollients to restore and maintain skin integrity. *Nursing Standard* **22**(41): 51–57.

Index